The CBT
Good Habit
Journal

Teach Yourself®

The CBT
Good Habit
Journal

A mindful journal for replacing anxiety
and stress with clarity and calm

Gill Hasson and Christine Wilding

First published in Great Britain in 2018 by John Murray Learning. An Hachette UK company.

British Library Cataloguing in Publication Data: a catalogue record for this title is available from the British Library.

Library of Congress Catalog Card Number: on file.

ISBN: 978 1 4736 5789 2

2

The publisher has used its best endeavours to ensure that any website addresses referred to in this book are correct and active at the time of going to press. However, the publisher and the author have no responsibility for the websites and can make no guarantee that a site will remain live or that the content will remain relevant, decent or appropriate.

The publisher has made every effort to mark as such all words which it believes to be trademarks. The publisher should also like to make it clear that the presence of a word in the book, whether marked or unmarked, in no way affects its legal status as a trademark.

Every reasonable effort has been made by the publisher to trace the copyright holders of material in this book. Any errors or omissions should be notified in writing to the publisher, who will endeavour to rectify the situation for any reprints and future editions.

This book is for information or educational purposes only and is not intended to act as a substitute for medical advice or treatment. Any person with a condition requiring medical attention should consult a qualified medical practitioner or suitable therapist.

Illustrations © Melissa Baker

Typeset by Cenveo® Publisher Services.

Printed and bound in Great Britain by CPI Group (UK) Ltd., Croydon, CR0 4YY.

John Murray Learning policy is to use papers that are natural, renewable and recyclable products and made from wood grown in sustainable forests. The logging and manufacturing processes are expected to conform to the environmental regulations of the country of origin.

Carmelite House

50 Victoria Embankment

London EC4Y 0DZ

www.hodder.co.uk

Contents

Introduction

Are you someone who spends quite a bit of time trying to work out how you can feel better about yourself, other people or the world around you? Perhaps you think that if you could only get your life into better shape all would be well?

Yet the most contented and well-adjusted among us are not always those who have the talent and skills, the nicest friends and family, the best job or ideal lifestyle. Those people often have difficulties in their lives too. So how do they – and how can you – learn to feel good whatever the circumstances?

Feeling good and feeling better start with accepting a basic truth: happiness is dependent not on what happens but on our **thoughts** about what happens.

This is the premise of cognitive behavioural therapy – **CBT**. CBT focuses not on what happens to us but on how we think about what happens to us and how we behave as a result of the way we think. It takes a look at whether our thinking and behaviours are helping our situation or keeping us stuck, or even making things worse. And, if our thinking and behaviours are not helpful, CBT looks at how best we can change what we think and do.

CBT shows you how to embrace new thinking and behaviour: ways of thinking and behaving that don't always seem clear and obvious at the start but which can be life-changing once mastered. These new ways will become skills, things you can do well.

This book is going to help you to learn some good, basic skills that will stay with you for life. These skills will become habits – good habits!

How to use this journal

The CBT Good Habit Journal is a place for exploration, change and growth. Of course you can dip in and out of the book if you prefer, but the real benefit will come from starting at the beginning and working through, so that you can consistently build on your understanding, develop skills and establish good habits.

In this way the book is rather like a course you might take, giving you things to do that will raise your awareness and curiosity and help you to learn how to think and see things differently.

The exercises, activities, meditations, etc., throughout this book will enable you to understand, document and process your thoughts, feelings and experiences in a helpful and creative way.

As you progress through the journal you'll discover that, rather than letting thoughts and feelings swirl around in your head or stay bottled up inside, writing them down helps you to disentangle them and think in clearer, more helpful ways.

Although the exercises and activities ahead range from being interesting and challenging to whacky and fun, they are all serious in their intention to help you see yourself and your world in a different way – a more positive, happier way.

In an effort to change your mind and your habits for the better, do try to read, write, and do the exercises and activities from one or two pages of this book if not every day, then every few days. You'll likely miss days. That's ok. Commit to them again the next day. For the next few weeks, make *The CBT Good Habit Journal* one of your new good habits.

Get started now!

Chapter 1
Goals

Past goals

Here's a list of common goals. Tick any that you've achieved. Then add any other goals you can think of that you set yourself and have achieved.

☐ Learned to drive

☐ Visited a European city or a city in the USA

☐ Moved into a new home

☐ Got the job

☐ Got the place on a course

☐ Cleaned the kitchen

☐ Completed a charity challenge

☐ Decorated a room

☐

☐

☐

☐

☐

☐

☐

☐

☐

☐

☐

☐

'Would you tell me, please, which way I ought to go from here?' 'That depends a good deal on where you want to get to,' said the Cat. 'I don't much care where –' said Alice. 'Then it doesn't matter which way you go,' said the Cat.

From *Alice's Adventures in Wonderland* by Lewis Carroll.

The cat's advice to Alice underlines the importance of knowing where you want to go before you set off down any path.

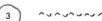

Having goals to aim for

In order to work with CBT you need something specific to work towards: a situation you want to change for the better or something you would like the confidence to be able to do. You need a goal.

Having goals you want to achieve can give you a positive path to follow. As you achieve each goal you create the momentum that helps you to develop good, helpful habits.

Think about what it is that you would like this book to help you achieve – perhaps within a month, three months, six months or a year's time. Ask yourself 'What do I want to achieve?' or 'How do I want things to be different?' 'What do I want to be able to do but don't yet have the confidence?'

You may already know what you want to change and work towards achieving. Here are some ideas:

☐ Change my job
☐ Learn a new skill
☐ Feel better about myself
☐ Stand up to a difficult person
☐ Be less anxious
☐ Run a marathon
☐ Ask for a pay rise
☐ Sign up to a class or join a club
☐ Take part in a sport
☐ Join a choir or a theatre company
☐ Have friends round for dinner
☐ Give a speech or presentation

☐ Go on a trip, by car, train or bus
☐ Work freelance
☐ Run my own business
☐ Return to study
☐ Declutter my home
☐ Leave a job, university course, relationship or friendship
☐ Write a book
☐ Enter a talent show
☐ Make new friends
☐ Travel abroad
☐ Clean the kitchen
☐ Be more fit and healthy
☐ Earn more money

Goals

Whatever it is you want to do or change for the better, write down your goal or goals here.

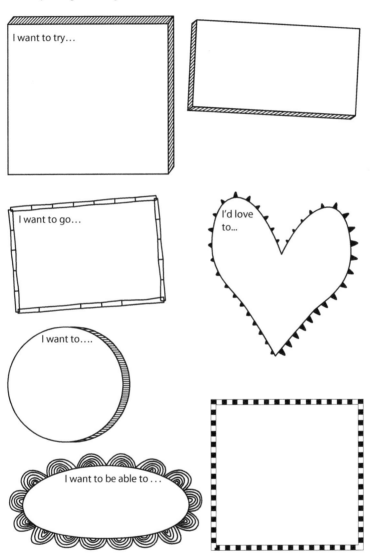

I want to try…

I want to go…

I'd love to…

I want to….

I want to be able to . . .

Be specific

Is your goal (or goals) specific? If your goal is to be happier, start by choosing a specific situation that you want to be happier in. Is your goal to travel somewhere? Where? When? If you want to be less anxious or be able to cope better in social situations, choose a specific situation in which you want to be less anxious or more at ease. Do you want to change your job? To do what? To work freelance? To set up your own company?

If your goal is an issue or problem that you want to deal with, think about what the result or outcome will be once the problem has been solved. What do you see yourself doing?

The more specific your goals are, the more likely you are to achieve them. Write down your specific goal or goals.

Goal:

Specific goal:

Goal:

Specific goal:

Goal:

Specific goal:

Set your goal as a positive statement

To increase your chances of achieving your goal, you'll need to think of it in positive terms. Goals that are framed in terms such as 'don't' 'mustn't', 'can't', or 'won't', 'shouldn't' or 'stop,' 'lose' or 'quit' are not so likely to motivate you.

Negative goal

→ I don't want to be working in this company anymore.

→ I want to stop feeling so anxious.

Positive goal

→ I want to have found a new job by the end of the year.

→ I want to feel calmer and more confident in a variety of situations.

Are your goals framed in positive terms? If not, rewrite them.

Negative goal

→

→

→

→

Positive goal

→

→

→

→

Goals framed in positive terms tell you what to do rather than what not to do. Thinking like this creates a positive attitude instead of feelings of struggle.

Why?

Write down why you want to achieve a goal. Why is it important to you? What do you hope to gain by achieving each goal?

Goal:

Reason to achieve the goal;

Goal:

Reason to achieve the goal;

Goal:

Reason to achieve the goal;

Goal:

Reason to achieve the goal;

Goal:

Reason to achieve the goal;

Where to start?

If you have several goals, which one do you want to work on first? A good way to decide is to give each goal a value rating between 1 and 10. If it's urgent and important give it a 10. Rate the other goals according to how urgent and/or important they are to you.

You can give your goal a further rating according to how hard you think it will be to achieve. Rate the goals from 1–10, where 1 is 'Hard to achieve' and 10 is 'Easier to achieve'.

Goal:

Urgent/important:

How hard or easy to achieve:

Goal:

Urgent/important:

How hard or easy to achieve:

Goal:

Urgent/important:

How hard or easy to achieve:

Goal:

Urgent/important:

How hard or easy to achieve:

How it works

Deadlines

Don't I have to decide when I need to achieve my goals?

Knowing when you want to achieve something by helps focus your efforts, but it's best not to become too concerned with having a deadline.

Pressure can be positive and motivating, but it can also create stress. If you don't meet the deadline or reach your target, you risk feeling like you failed. Instead of giving yourself a deadline to reach, simply focus on working consistently towards what it is you want to achieve, one step at a time.

But I do have a deadline - I've got to give a presentation to some clients next week

Of course, some goals have an inherent deadline; if you have a presentation that you have to give in two weeks' time you can't change that date! What you can still do though, is take things step by step – knowing that you *can* make progress – rather than having the pressure of a deadline looming towards you.

Really? CBT can help me even in a short time period? That sounds like hard work!

Whatever it is you want to be able to do with CBT, although it may present a challenge it doesn't have to be too difficult. What could feel impossible in one giant leap, becomes a lot more doable as a series of smaller steps. CBT breaks things down into smaller more achievable steps. Taking a step-by-step approach is the most positive way forward because it means you set yourself up for constant successes by achieving small targets along the way.

CBT is not a quick fix, but the more you practise the techniques, the sooner you'll progress.

No matter how many mistakes you make or how slow you progress, you're still way ahead of anyone who isn't trying.

Tony Robbins

Step by step

To achieve any goal, you will need to break down the task into a series of smaller steps. Following a recipe to produce a dish is a good example of this. Try this recipe:

Lemon posset

Lemon posset can be made in five steps.

Ingredients:
600ml double cream
200g golden caster sugar
zest 3 lemons, plus 75ml juice

(1) **Put the cream in a big saucepan with the sugar and gently heat, stirring, until the sugar has melted.**

(2) **Bring to a simmer and, stirring all the time, allow to gently bubble for one minute.**

(3) **Turn off the heat and stir in the lemon zest and juice.**

(4) **Divide between pots or bowls. Cool to room temperature.**

(5) **Cover and chill for at least three hours.**

Favourite recipe

Write down one of your favourite recipes here.

Step 1:

Step 2:

Step 3:

Step 4:

Step 5:

It might look like a long list, but each step of the recipe you complete is one step closer to the finished dish.

Past goals

Choose a past goal that you achieved.

What was the very first thing you did? What was the first step you took? And the next? And the next? And after that?

Goal achieved:

First step:

Second step:

Third step:

Fourth step:

Fifth step:

Sixth step:

Doing things one step at a time also gives you a chance to look at what is working and what isn't, and to decide if you need to change tactics. So, as you go through this book, review your outcomes. What worked? What helped and went well? What didn't work? What needs adjusting? Use the space below for your notes.

How it works

Imagine it

How can visualizing myself achieving my goals help me?

If you can imagine yourself achieving something, your brain then believes and accepts it *is* indeed possible and that you can do it. The future you see is the future you get. If you constantly visualize not being able to do something, your brain believe and accepts that too.

See yourself achieving whatever it is you want to do, be or get. Think about how you'll feel when you achieve that goal and how pleased you'll be with yourself and what you've achieved. Return to that image and feeling whenever you are unsure and feel your confidence slipping.

Good habit

Get into the habit of visualizing yourself doing and achieving whatever it is you're aiming for.

Draw a picture of yourself doing whatever it is you hope to do: achieving one of your goals.

30-second meditation

Sit or stand up straight in a comfortable position. Breathe in, breathe out. Pause. One more time, this time a little slower and deeper: breathe in, breathe out.

You just did a mini-meditation.

Remember

o In order to work with CBT and form good habits you need something specific to work towards. You need a goal. Ask yourself, 'What do I want to achieve?', 'What do I want the confidence to be able to do?' or 'How do I want things to be different?'

o The more specific your goals are, the more likely you are to achieve them.

o Think of your goal in positive terms. Goals framed in positive terms tell you what to do rather than what not to do.

o If you have several goals, decide which one you want to work on first. A good way to prioritize things is to give each goal a value rating between 1 and 5.

o Instead of giving yourself a deadline to reach, simply focus on working consistently, step by step towards what it is you want to achieve.

o Any goal you've achieved in the past has been the result of a series of steps.

o If you can imagine yourself achieving something, your brain then believes and accepts it *is* indeed possible and that you *can* do it.

Chapter 2

Being aware of your thoughts

What are you thinking?

During the next 24 hours, check in with your thinking from time to time. Write down, for example, what your thoughts are about the day ahead when you wake up. Then, set an alarm on your phone to remind you to write down your thoughts at five different times during the day.

Time:

Thought:

Who or what the thought was about:

Time:

Thought:

Who or what the thought was about:

Time:

Thought:

Who or what the thought was about:

Time:

Thought:

Who or what the thought was about:

Time:

Thought:

Who or what the thought was about:

Time:

Thought:

Who or what the thought was about:

Good habit

Get into the habit of noticing your thoughts. You can use a 'mindfulness bell' app on your phone or computer, a note on a computer screen or a screen saver that simply asks 'Thinking...?'

Rubin's vase

Look at this image. Do you see a vase or two faces?

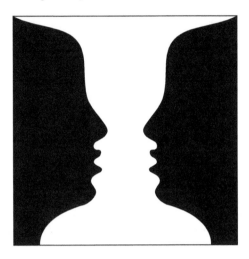

Either way of seeing is true and real. But what makes one more real than the other is simply the one that in any given moment you can see. It's not possible to see both images at the same time – in seeing one image, your mind excludes the possibility of seeing the other image. To see the alternative image you have to refocus.

As with seeing, it's much the same with thinking – there's more than one way of interpreting or thinking about things. And when your thoughts are fixed in one way, it's not easy to think in a different way.

How it works

Self-talk

Is my mind always thinking?

Pretty much, yes. In any one day we all have many, many thoughts. Our thoughts automatically enter our mind and provide us with a running commentary rather like a radio that is permanently tuned to a talk station.

Your self-talk – your thoughts – direct your actions and behaviour. Some of your thoughts may be positive and constructive: thinking about how to help someone; working out a solution to a problem; looking forward to an event; remembering something good that happened.

Other thoughts will be neutral thoughts: observations and acknowledgements of day-to-day events; for example 'It's raining, I'll need an umbrella'.

Negative thoughts interpret ideas or events in a pessimistic way, for example: 'This is never going to work out'; 'Why does this happen to me?'; 'They'll think I'm stupid'; 'It's not fair'.

Thinking: the talking of the soul with itself.

Plato

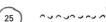

Walking commentary meditation

Plan a five-minute walk – in the park, round the block, along a footpath, up the road and back again or wherever. Once you set off, begin a running commentary in your head describing your walk and everything you notice. For example, 'I'm opening the door. I'm leaving the house. I'm shutting the door. I'm walking down the path and I'm turning left. A car just drove past. I'm walking past my neighbours' house. I can hear the birds singing ...'

Notice you are simply *describing* what you are doing and what you are experiencing – what you see, hear smell etc. You are not making judgements. Nothing is good or bad. Your thoughts are neutral.

Glass of water

Is the glass half full or half empty?

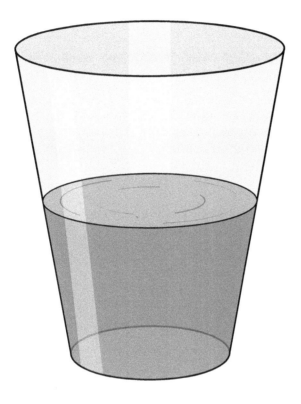

If you think the glass is half empty then you're likely to be a negative thinker. If you see the glass as half full, you're more likely to be a positive thinker. Neither negative thinking nor positive thinking is more real or true than the other. Either way of thinking could be real or true. But what makes one way of thinking more real is the one you think and believe to be true.

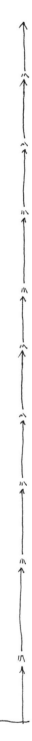

Is your thinking open or closed?

Try to be honest with your answers in this quiz: even though you may be able to guess what the 'correct' answer is, try to go with your instinctive response.

1. **You are thinking about New Year's resolutions. Are you more likely to:**

   a) Feel that you *ought* to make resolutions and come up with one or two.
   b) Make a resolution or two and plan how you will achieve your goals.

2. **You don't like your job and you're beginning to dread going in. Are you more likely to:**

   a) Start suffering from headaches or stomach problems and regularly take days off sick.
   b) Tell yourself to 'Get a grip' and that 'Life is too short' and then start looking for another job.

3. **You want to get fitter. Are you more likely to:**

   a) Think to yourself 'I don't know where to start or how to get more fit' and feel helpless.
   b) Plan how to include more exercise in your daily routine.

4. **A friend texts you to say there's nothing to worry about but they need to speak with you about something. Are you more likely to think:**

   a) 'I bet there **is** something to worry about. I wonder what's wrong or what I've done wrong?'
   b) 'I wonder what this might be about?'

5. You have to pull out of going to an important event with a friend. Are you more likely to:

   a) Feel guilty and avoid your friend until you think she's forgotten about it.
   b) Feel guilty but think of a way to make it up to her in the next week or two.

6. You are driving your car and you run out of petrol. Your partner used the car before you. Are you more likely to:

   a) Blame your partner. They *knew* you needed the car today.
   b) Be angry and think 'D'oh! How could I not have checked the fuel gauge before I set off?'

7. You have moved to a different area, but you're finding it difficult to settle. Do you:

   a) Keep it to yourself as you don't want to admit you may have made a mistake. Tell yourself you've been stupid and feel more and more miserable.
   b) Give yourself more time. Decide to find a way to get involved with the local community and start to feel more cheerful about the possibilities.

8. You discover that a friend has lied to you recently. Are you more likely to:

   a) Feel upset and angry, have sleepless nights worrying about what you should do, but not say anything. Instead talk about it with a different friend (who you know doesn't like this friend) to confirm that your lying friend is a bitch.
   b) Feel upset and angry, talk to your friend and ask them for an explanation.

9. You are interviewed for a job that you would like, but you don't get it. Are you more likely to:

   a) Feel disappointed and blame the interviewer for not knowing how to carry out a fair interview.
   b) Feel disappointed but ask for feedback and use that feedback to help you with the next interview.

10. In the last week your television, washing machine and computer have all broken down. Are you more likely to:

    a) Feel overwhelmed and complain how unfair and stressful your life is.
    b) Think through how you can best pay for everything – what could be repaired, or bought second hand, and what has to be replaced with a new model?

11. You go out with friends on a week night. When you finally get to bed are you more likely to think:

    a) I'm annoyed with myself for having stayed out too late; I've got work in the morning.
    b) I've had such a fun time!

12. The day before you go on holiday, are you more likely to:

    a) Keep thinking you might forget something and find it difficult to get to sleep.
    b) Be excited and can't wait to leave.

13. **You have the opportunity to apply for a promotion/go on a blind date/travel somewhere new. You think:**

a) I'm not doing it. It'll probably all turn out badly.
b) I'll give it a go and see how it turns out. Nothing ventured, nothing gained!

The more often you answered a) the more areas of your life could benefit from CBT.

Notice how a) answers all reflect the narrow thinking that contracts your world and limits your opportunities and possibilities; b) answers on the other hand, all reflect thinking that opens up possibilities and opportunities for you.

Superstitions

Which, if any, of these superstitions do you believe?

- ☐ Friday the 13th is unlucky.
- ☐ Washing your car will bring rain.
- ☐ You'll have seven years of bad luck if you break a mirror.
- ☐ If you make a funny face and the wind changes you'll stay looking that way.
- ☐ It's bad luck to open an umbrella indoors, put shoes on a table or cross on the stairs.
- ☐ If you can blow out all the candles on your birthday cake in one go you'll get whatever you wish for.
- ☐ Bad luck comes in threes.
- ☐ A cat has nine lives.
- ☐ Wear your lucky underwear and you'll do well in the game, interview or exam.

From a rational point of view, there is no logical connection between one event – putting shoes on a table, for example – and what happens next.

You may not believe in any of these superstitions and think that anyone who does is ridiculous. Yet, when it comes to your own thoughts, you probably believe they are all rational and valid. It rarely occurs to us that our thoughts about events might be illogical, unreasonable or even just plain unhelpful!

One of the difficulties in recognizing negative thoughts is that they are very good at appearing, on the face of things, to be rational truths. Because of this we rarely question them and simply 'go along' with them.

The problem is, many of our thoughts and beliefs can distort and twist events in ways that can upset, disturb and distress us.

Superstition brings bad luck.

Paul Carvel

Finish the sentence

Finish this sentence.

If something can go wrong …
   a) … it probably will.
   b) … it can also go right.

For there is nothing either good or bad, but thinking
makes it so.

Shakespeare

Different interpretations

Rumours have been going around the workplace that redundancies are soon to be announced. Ali, Nik and Sara each have different thoughts about the possibility of losing their job.

> Ali: I think I'll make a list of contacts, agencies and companies and see what possibilities there might be.

> Nik: I'm sure they'll want to get rid of me. I'm not the best at this job – there're others they'll want to keep on. I can't see how I'm going to get another job.

> Sara: It's bound to be me. Last in first out. It's not fair. I knew I should never have taken this job – I should've stayed in my old job.

Nik and Sara become stuck in their ways of thinking about the possible redundancies. Nik and Sara's thoughts limit and narrow their opportunities and choices. Their negative thinking creates a spiral of unhelpful thoughts and difficult feelings.

Ali's thinking reflects an open mind and opens up his ideas, thoughts and actions. His positive thinking brings hope; that events **can** turn out for the best.

How it works

Positive thinking

So think positive and life will always be good?
Having a positive optimistic outlook doesn't mean that you always feel good and happy. People who are positive still have worries, feel sad, disappointed, guilty or angry and so on.

But their positive outlook prevents them from getting stuck in unhelpful thoughts and enables them to manage difficulties in a way that doesn't drag them down even further. Is that it?
Yes. Hopeful, optimistic thoughts can expand your world and the possibilities in it. They can open your mind, which in turn allows you to see more possibilities and options in a range of situations.

In contrast, narrowed thinking focuses your attention on a situation so that it becomes the **only** thing you can think about. Often, this can be a good thing. It might not feel nice but 'negative', narrow thoughts can prompt you to take focused, positive action. If, for example, you were worried about missing your flight, you'd constantly check the departures board; your mind would focus in on the departures board; you'd be unlikely to think of anything else.

In other situations, negative thoughts can narrow and distort your world, keeping you feeling bad and leaving you stuck.

Anything and everything can be explained in both positive and negative ways. Negative thoughts interpret ideas or events in a pessimistic way and can cause you to feel anxious or scared, resentful and so on. Positive thoughts can positively influence how you feel and how you respond to situations and prompt you to feel happy.

I'd rather have a mind opened by wonder than one closed by belief.

Gerry Spence

Recognizing patterns

For each line of shapes, colour in the two shapes that will correctly complete the sequence.

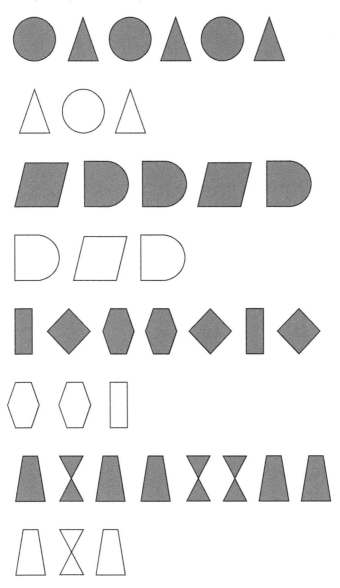

It wasn't difficult to complete these patterns, was it? CBT can help you recognize your own patterns - repeated ways - of thinking and behaving.

How it works

What are cognitive distortions?

You may have a tendency to fall into particular patterns of unhelpful thinking. These patterns are often referred to as 'cognitive distortions'. Here are some examples.

Confirmation bias

Confirmation bias involves looking for and accepting evidence to confirm what you've already decided is true.

Jumping to a conclusion

This involves deciding something is true without having all the relevant information.

Tunnel thinking

Imagine looking down a cardboard tube. What can you see? Or rather, what can't you see? With tunnel thinking, you are blind to other possibilities and options. Instead of seeing the whole picture, you focus on the negative aspects of a situation.

Polarized thinking

It's 'all or nothing' thinking. There's no middle ground. Things are good or bad, right or wrong, a success or a total failure. There's no room for mistakes and no room for improvement.

Catastrophizing

When you catastrophize, you think the absolute worst is going to happen in a situation.

Mind reading

With mind reading, you believe you know what the other person is thinking and that their thoughts and intentions are negative.

Blaming

This involves placing all responsibility for something that's gone wrong on someone else or something else. Alternatively, you might place all the blame on yourself if things don't turn out well. Rightly or wrongly you may feel responsible for the wellbeing of others and the way events turn out.

Cognitive distortions can easily convince you that your thoughts *are* rational and true. But actually they limit your options, influence the way you behave and make you feel bad about the world, other people, yourself and your abilities.

Study the hurtful patterns of your life. Then don't repeat them.

Yasmin Mogahed

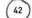

Spot the cognitive distortions

Match the cognitive distortions in the scenarios below. Which cognitive distortion is happening in which scenario?

1. Jumping to conclusions

2. Mind reading

3. Confirmation bias

4. Tunnel thinking

5. Catastrophizing

6. Blaming

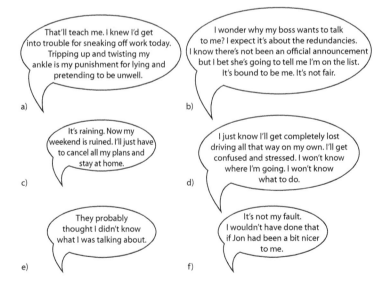

a) That'll teach me. I knew I'd get into trouble for sneaking off work today. Tripping up and twisting my ankle is my punishment for lying and pretending to be unwell.

b) I wonder why my boss wants to talk to me? I expect it's about the redundancies. I know there's not been an official announcement but I bet she's going to tell me I'm on the list. It's bound to be me. It's not fair.

c) It's raining. Now my weekend is ruined. I'll just have to cancel all my plans and stay at home.

d) I just know I'll get completely lost driving all that way on my own. I'll get confused and stressed. I won't know where I'm going. I won't know what to do.

e) They probably thought I didn't know what I was talking about.

f) It's not my fault. I wouldn't have done that if Jon had been a bit nicer to me.

(Answers at the back of the book.)

Identifying your thought patterns

Can you recognize any of your own negative thought patterns? Try and remember some difficult stressful events and situations you recently experienced. Maybe you lost something? Did someone criticize you or let you down badly? Perhaps you had a long travel delay? Write down which thoughts may have been examples of cognitive distortions.

Tunnel thinking:

Catastrophizing:

Blaming:

Jumping to conclusions:

Mind reading:

Confirmation bias:

How it works

Habits

How are habits formed?

Imagine you are walking through a field of long grass. The grass is so long that you have to tread it down as you walk to the other side of the field. The next day, you retrace your steps and walk across the field again. This time it's a little easier. Over the next few days and weeks you walk exactly the same path across the field – it becomes so well worn that you walk the path automatically; you don't have to think about it.

What's this got to do with how habits are formed?

The process of establishing a path through a field and automatically walking along it is similar to how the neural pathways in our brain functions.

When we think or do something for the first time, nerve cells are activated and a new neural pathway is created. Then, each time we think or behave in that same way, our brain uses that same neural pathway. The pathway becomes stronger and stronger each time it's used. It's just like walking through a field of long grass, the more often that path is trodden, the more established the path becomes and the more likely it is that we'll take that path.

This means that if we do something often enough, it becomes automatic. The things we do on a daily basis – brushing our teeth, driving, texting, etc. – we do so often that our brain uses the same neural pathways and we don't have to think about them.

However, as well as establishing helpful ways of doing and thinking things, the processes of neural pathways can establish behaviour habits that are not so good for us; smoking for example.

If we often interpret events in a negative way, then we create strong negative neural pathways in our brain. Those neural pathways can become so established that they also become habits; negative thinking habits.

So if we know that doing something regularly makes it more likely we'll continue doing it, why don't we just stop doing it?

Your thoughts and reactions to events are so powerful *because* you rarely have conscious awareness or control over them. Your mind simply accepts everything it's 'told' and you respond accordingly.

If you're more inclined to think negatively, your brain will automatically use negative neural pathways and you will interpret events in negative ways. On the other hand, if you're more inclined to positive thinking, your brain will interpret and make sense of events in positive ways. And, whichever way you're inclined to think, each time you do so, you reinforce that particular way of thinking, interpreting and explaining things.

Even when you become aware of your negative thinking habit, like all habits, it can be a real struggle to break it.

What's the good news?

The good news is that your way of interpreting events does not have to be permanent. You *can* overcome negative thinking. You *can* learn to think in a more positive, helpful way. You have to make a conscious effort – commit to change and practising those changes with deliberate effort.

Once you begin to change how you think or what you do, then new, positive neural pathways are formed. When you continue using these new positive pathways, they become stronger and deeper. Eventually, they will replace the old ways of thinking and behaving. You will have rewired – or reprogrammed – your brain.

Identifying the strongest thoughts

One way to identify why you're thinking and feeling like you do is to ask yourself, 'Why does that matter?'

For example, imagine a friend cancels your evening out together. Your immediate thought is:

Oh great. Now I'm not going out tonight.

Why does this matter?

I was looking forward to an evening with my friend

Why does that matter?

I haven't been out for ages

Why does that matter?

Colleagues at work are always talking about where they've been and what they've done. I've got nothing to talk about.

Why does that matter?

I feel left out.

Why does that matter?

I've got no friends. I feel pathetic.

Now you have your strong 'causal' thought: the thought that creates the physical feelings, behaviour and emotions. Recognizing the significant thought is helpful to overcoming the negativity it creates.

Animal mind

If your mind was an animal right now, what would it be?

→ An owl – calm and wise

→ A monkey – chattering and swinging from one tree to another

→ A parrot – squawking the same words and phrases over and over

→ An elephant – not forgetting

→ A frog – hopping around

→ A dolphin – graceful and agile

→ A bee – buzzing about

→ A tortoise – slow and deliberate

→ A butterfly – flitting around

Thinking about your own thinking

If you've read the last few pages then you've been thinking about your own thinking – a process known as 'meta cognition' from the Greek word *meta* meaning 'beyond or after'.

'Meta cognition' means you're taking a step beyond yourself and your thoughts so that you can look back and try to understand them.

Good habit

Get used to observing, say, the first three thoughts you have upon waking every day – were they ordinary neutral thoughts, positive thoughts or were they judgemental, anxious, apprehensive or blaming?

Start a habit of noticing a thought rather than believing it.

Positive word search

Find the words listed below, hidden in this word search. The words may read up, down, forward, backwards or diagonally.

```
t  f  f  l  x  d  l  l  w  h  w  w  u  l  c
u  m  b  m  k  u  s  u  j  a  s  h  j  i  r
l  m  z  n  f  a  p  f  e  p  m  u  t  n  y
u  c  a  e  m  h  p  p  w  p  b  s  k  x  c
g  t  p  k  j  k  p  l  g  y  i  z  i  v  v
s  o  f  d  d  d  x  e  i  m  x  d  i  z  j
h  r  e  k  u  u  u  h  i  p  z  p  y  p  y
c  j  g  d  o  u  y  t  p  m  o  i  l  z  x
z  y  o  p  c  u  p  w  c  s  f  x  j  f  c
r  o  a  r  t  o  j  j  i  s  t  r  o  n  g
g  l  e  k  e  p  m  t  u  o  x  b  k  q  h
m  r  y  r  a  z  i  k  i  n  d  n  e  s  s
m  r  k  j  t  v  f  m  n  d  m  p  v  k  l
t  q  a  i  e  o  b  x  l  a  r  k  g  y  p
t  r  u  s  t  k  a  s  m  k  h  i  w  b  e
```

good

happy

helpful

hopeful

kindness

optimistic

positive

strong

trust

Everyday meditation

Everyday routine tasks – washing up, cooking and cleaning – can help *challenge your thoughts, beliefs and assumptions* about what is a satisfying activity and what is a tedious chore.

Washing up is just washing up. Doing the laundry is just doing the laundry. Cleaning the bathroom is just cleaning the bathroom. None of these activities are good or bad. They're just activities. They're only difficult, boring, or something to be resented if you think of them in that way.

If cooking and cleaning seem like boring chores to you, try doing them as an exercise in mindfulness. Instead of the time being hurried and unpleasant, engage yourself with those tasks and do them well, without hurry.

Mindful washing up

Turn the water on, watch it flow from the taps and fill up the sink. Squirt the washing up liquid into the water and watch the bubbles form. Feel the warmth of the water, the texture of the dish cloth.

Pick up the first plate, and feel its weight in your hands. Take your time washing each piece of crockery and cutlery, each pot and pan. At some point, your mind will wander and your thoughts will intrude, telling you to get a move on, prompting you to think about other things. That's ok. Each time you notice your thoughts are wandering, simply return your thoughts to what you are doing now, at this moment.

Consider the marvel of indoor plumbing; the privilege of hot and cold running water. Appreciate the simple pleasure that comes from having control of one small part of your world. If you're anxious, allow the ritual to calm you. If you're angry or frustrated, express your emotional energy by scrubbing pots and pans until they shine.

Remember

o In any one day we all have many, many thoughts which automatically enter our mind and provide us with a running commentary.

o There's more than one way of of thinking about things. It is the way you think and what you believe to be true that makes one way of thinking more real than the other.

o It rarely occurs to us that our thoughts about events might be illogical, unreasonable or even just unhelpful.

o You may have a tendency to fall into particular patterns of negative thinking. These patterns are often referred to as 'cognitive distortions'.

o Cognitive distortions can narrow your thoughts in ways that contract and distort your world, upset, disturb and distress you and keep you feeling bad.

o In contrast, in a range of situations, hopeful optimistic thoughts open your mind, which in turn allows you to see more possibilities and options.

o The good news is that your way of interpreting events does not have to be permanent and your outlook is not fixed. You can overcome negative thinking. You can learn to think in a more positive, helpful way.

o Once you begin to change how you think or what you do, then new, positive neural pathways are formed. When you continue using these new positive pathways, they become stronger and deeper. Eventually, they will replace the old ways of thinking and behaving. You will have rewired – or reprogrammed – your brain!

Chapter 3

Challenging negative thinking, and finding alternative ways of thinking

Pink flamingo

Picture a pink flamingo. A pretty, elegant bird.

Now, for the next minute try **not** to think of a pink flamingo –
block out any thoughts of a pink flamingo.

After one minute, turn the page.

Thought changing - not thought stopping

How did you get on? Not easy was it?

So how can you stop thoughts entering your head? And how can you stop *negative* thoughts entering your head?

Rather than spend time and energy trying to **stop** negative thoughts, CBT encourages you to **change** your thoughts.

What a liberation to know that the 'voice in my head' is not who I am. Who am I then? The one who sees that.

Elkhart Tolle

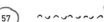

Thought record

Here's an example of a person's thinking. Below, write down your own examples of events that have wound you up (at work, in public or with friends or family) and the thoughts that you had – or were likely to have had – at the time.

Situation: What happened?

I got turned down for a place on a course.

Thoughts: What went through my mind?

No point even going for the interviews at the other universities – they'll turn me down too.

Situation: What happened?

Thoughts: What went through my mind?

Situation: What happened?

Thoughts: What went through my mind?

Situation: What happened?

Thoughts: What went through my mind?

Thoughts about your goals

Go back to the goals you wrote down in Chapter 1. On this page, write down each goal again. For each goal, complete a sentence beginning with the word 'but'.

Goal:

To have friends round for dinner

Thought:

but I'm not a good cook.

Goal:

Thought:

but

Goal:

Thought:

but

Goal:

Thought:

but

Five things I know for sure

Write down five things you know or think about yourself, life and other people.

1

2

3

4

5

Now tick which facts you are 100 per cent sure about. Put a star * next to any facts you're not 100 per cent certain of.

There are no facts, only interpretations.

Friedrich Nietzsche

Music meditation

Listen to music differently. With a 'beginner's mind' you can listen to familiar pieces of music as if for the first time. Choose a favourite piece of music. Pick out an element that you don't usually listen to – the beat, the melody, the lyrics or a particular instrument. Now listen to and follow the music, focusing on the new element you have chosen. Even though you have listened to this piece of music many times before, when you listen with a 'beginner's mind', you experience it anew.

Are you certain?

How can you be certain that anything you think or believe is true? There's more than one way of thinking about yourself, other people and the world. What you don't want to do though, is to start arguing with yourself. Telling yourself you're 'wrong' to think the way you do won't work. You won't win!

You can challenge your thoughts by asking yourself questions that can help you recognize that there is more than one way to think about things. Go back to your 'but' thoughts on page 59. These are likely to be negative thoughts. Write them out below, then rate how strongly you believe each thought on a scale of 1-10, where 1 is 'Not really' and 10 is 'Very much'.

Negative thought:

On a scale of 1-10 how certain am I?

How do I know this thought is true? What evidence do I have?

Negative thought:

On a scale of 1-10 how certain am I?

How do I know this thought is true? What evidence do I have?

Challenging negative thoughts

Challenging your thoughts can help you to see whether your view is reasonable and helpful. Think about in what way your thoughts did or didn't help each situation. Read back over your thoughts on pages 58 and 59 and for each thought, answer the following questions:

Thought:

Is this thought helping me?

Yes. How?

No. Why?

Discover that your thoughts are just words and sounds. Take one of your negative unhelpful thoughts and type it into Google translate. Choose another language to translate it into. Read and listen to the translation.

Nursery rhymes

Singing unhelpful thoughts to the tunes of nursery rhymes helps to defuse the thoughts – to weaken them.

Write down one of your negative thoughts then sing it to the tune of one or more of these nursery rhymes and children's songs.

Thought:

- ☐ Hickory Dickory Dock
- ☐ The Wheels on the Bus
- ☐ Round and Round the Garden
- ☐ Humpty Dumpty
- ☐ Row Row Row Your Boat
- ☐ Ring a Ring a Roses
- ☐ Twinkle Twinkle Little Star
- ☐ Incy Wincy Spider
- ☐ Old MacDonald
- ☐ *Postman Pat* theme

good habit

Get into the habit of challenging your thoughts. When you notice that negative thoughts are entering your mind, say 'stop!' to yourself. If you're alone, you can say it out loud, but it's also effective when you just say it in your head.

Get used to the idea of stopping to challenge your thinking when you recognize negative thinking: when you're feeling anxious, blaming, irritated, frustrated, jealous, or guilty etc.

Images can help: try imagining a bright red stop sign that you picture in your mind's eye when intrusive thoughts begin to appear.

Remember

o Rather than spend time and energy trying to simply *stop* negative thoughts, CBT encourages you to *change* your thoughts.

o You can challenge your mind's negative automatic thoughts by asking yourself questions that can help you recognize that there is more than one way to think about things.

A different way of thinking

Becoming aware of and challenging your thoughts is the first step towards learning to think in a more helpful, positive way. The next step is to see if there's a different way of thinking about a situation – a more helpful way.

Grandma is sitting in her chair knitting but her two-year-old granddaughter Ella is disturbing her by playing with the ball of wool. Ella's Dad suggests putting Ella in the playpen. But Ella's Mum suggests it would make more sense to put Grandma in the playpen. It's a different way of thinking.

Lateral thinking

The cake

Can you think of a way to cut a cake into eight equal pieces with only three cuts? There is more than one way.

(Answers at the back of the book.)

The bus stop

You're driving in your car on a stormy night, when you pass by a bus stop and you see three people waiting for the bus:

a) A frail old lady
b) Your best friend
c) The perfect partner you have been waiting for all your life

Knowing that there can only be one passenger in your car, who would you choose? You want to help everyone out but your car can only take one passenger, so who should it be?

(Answer at the back of the book.)

How it works

Confirmation bias

You drive into a car park looking for a space. Do you notice all the red cars or all the spaces?

You return to the car park. You're looking for your car. It's a red car. Are you likely to notice all the car parking spaces or the red cars?

Is finding a parking space and a red car what's known as 'the law of attraction'?

Not exactly. When you drove into the car park, your brain and all your senses were already primed to notice a parking space, not a red car. But when you returned to the car park, your brain and all your senses were expecting to notice a red car, not a parking space. There's nothing magical about it; your mind simply notices and pays attention to what it's hoping and expecting to find; what it thinks is likely to happen.

What's that got to do with negative, unhelpful thinking?

Just as it's easier to notice a parking space when you're looking for one than it is a red car (and vice versa), it's often much easier to find evidence to support a negative view than it is to find any against it. This is due to negative thinking bias, meaning that if you're in a low mood or you feel pessimistic, your thinking leans that way and you don't see alternatives.

So what's going on in my head?

You have a system in your brain called the 'reticular activating system (RAS) that controls your consciousness. The RAS filters out everything that doesn't support your most prevalent thoughts and behaviour. So, your mind has a tendency, first and foremost, to notice and pay attention to experiences that match its pre-existing thoughts and beliefs.

Evidence to support an alternative view can often be outside of your awareness so you need to search hard for it.

It turns out confirmation bias means exactly what
I expected it to mean.

Moose Allain

 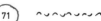

The house

As you read this story, underline anything you think might be of interest to an estate agent.

'Mum works all day on a Thursday so today is a good day for bunking off lessons,' said Al to his friend Josh. 'Let's go!' The two boys ran until they got to the driveway of the house. Tall hedges hid the house from the road – the boys slowed down and strolled across the large, pretty, front garden. 'I didn't know your house was this big,' said Josh. 'Yes, but it's nicer now since we had a conservatory built and a new stone fireplace put in,' replied Al.

There were front and back doors and a side door which led to the garage, which was empty except for three mountain bikes. They went into the house through the side door; Al explained that it was unlocked in case his younger sisters got home before their Mum. Josh wanted to see the house. Al started in the living room which had recently been redecorated. He put some music on and turned up the volume. 'Someone will hear us!' said Josh. 'No they won't,' said Al, 'the nearest neighbours are a quarter of a mile away.'

The formal dining room with all the bone china, silver and cut glass was no place to play and anyway, the boys were hungry. They went into the big, bright kitchen and raided the fridge for something to eat.

Al said they wouldn't bother going to the basement – it was damp and had a musty smell. Instead he took Josh to his Dad's study. 'This is where Dad keeps his signed photos of rock stars – Mick Jagger, David Bowie, The Beatles – and his rare coin collection,' said Al.

There were four bedrooms upstairs. Al showed Josh his Mum's *en suite* dressing room with its designer clothes and the locked box which held her jewellery. Then Al showed Josh his own room and pointed out the leak in the corner of the ceiling where the old roof had rotted. Finally they went into Al's big brother's room where they played on the games console for the next hour.

Now reread the story and underline anything you think might be of interest to a burglar. Notice how what is of interest to the burglar is different from what is of interest to the estate agent, and for what differing reasons.

If you change the way you look at things, the things you look at change.

Wayne Dyer

Change hands

Because of the interconnections between the nerve cells in your brain, when you think or do something new, you create new connections – neural pathways – in your brain. If your brain continues using these new pathways, they become stronger and deeper. Eventually, they will replace the old ways of thinking and behaving.

Using your non-dominant hand to perform a familiar task encourages your brain to create new neural pathways.

Hold a pen or pencil with your non-dominant hand and follow the instructions below, using the available space.

1. Draw a square.

2. Draw a circle.

3. Write the numbers 1 to 10.

4. Write your name.

5. Write the following: 'I'm writing this sentence with my non-dominant hand.'

Change hands

Use your non-dominant hand to do one of the following every day for a week or two. It will take time and effort, because the neural pathways for using your dominant hand are well established. But if you really want to do it, you can forge new neural pathways and develop the ability to do things with different hand. You can retrain your brain.

- Brush your teeth
- Make your tea or coffee
- Use a computer mouse
- Open doors

The same is true for anything you want to do or any way you would like to think: it takes effort and commitment, but it's not impossible and it's never too late!

Ask a friend

Collect alternative points of view. Ask two other people what they think about:

(1.) **The Royal Family**

Your thoughts:

First person's thoughts:

Second person's thoughts:

(2.) **Brussels sprouts**

Your thoughts:

First person's thoughts:

Second person's thoughts:

3. The Prime Minister

Your thoughts:

First person's thoughts:

Second person's thoughts:

4. Cats

Your thoughts:

First person's thoughts:

Second person's thoughts:

5. Coldplay

Your thoughts:

First person's thoughts:

Second person's thoughts:

6. Beards

Your thoughts:

First person's thoughts:

Second person's thoughts:

7. Online dating

Your thoughts:

First person's thoughts:

Second person's thoughts:

8. Living in the country

Your thoughts:

First person's thoughts:

Second person's thoughts:

9. Going to the gym

Your thoughts:

First person's thoughts:

Second person's thoughts:

10. Dark chocolate

Your thoughts:

First person's thoughts:

Second person's thoughts:

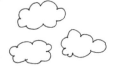

Alternative explanations

Challenging your negative thoughts interrupts them and stops them from snowballing. This frees you to start thinking and responding in more positive ways. Recognizing that the way you're thinking isn't helpful can prompt you to look at things differently. Here are some more questions to ask yourself:

1. How would a friend perceive this? What would they say to me?

2. If the situation was reversed, what positive things would I say to a friend?

3. What other explanations are there for what happened, is happening or could happen?

Change the script

Watch an episode of a soap opera or TV drama. Listen out for when a character says something negative. Then write an alternative sentence for that character.

Character:

What they said:

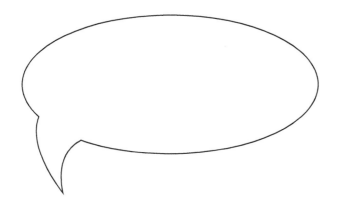

Alternative sentence:

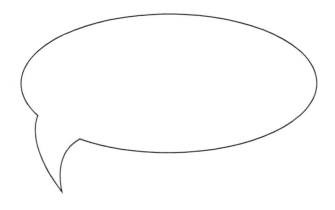

Tiny frogs

There was once a bunch of tiny frogs, who arranged a running competition. The goal was to run, hop and jump to the top of a very high tower. A big crowd gathered around the tower to see the race and cheer on the contestants.

The race began. No one in the crowd really believed that the tiny frogs would reach the top of the tower. They shouted, 'It's too difficult! They will NEVER make it to the top' and 'Not a chance. The tower is too high'.

The tiny frogs began collapsing, one by one except for a few who were managing to climb higher.

The crowd continued to yell, 'It's too difficult! It's much too hard! No one will make it!'

More tiny frogs got tired and gave up. But one continued higher and higher. This one wouldn't give up! And he reached the top.

Everyone wanted to know how this one frog managed such a great feat.

His secret? This little frog was deaf!

(Author Unknown)

It's not always possible or practical to completely withdraw from the negative people in your life. What you can do, however, is reduce the amount of time you spend around them and increase the amount of time you spend with positive people. These are people who make you laugh, people who have a positive outlook, people who encourage you.

Stay positive and happy. Work hard and don't give up hope. Be open to criticism and keep learning. Surround yourself with happy, warm and genuine people.

Tena Desae

Good habit

Identify and spend time with the positive people in your life

When you're stuck with unhelpful thoughts, seek out people who can put things into perspective and won't feed your negative thinking.

Which people come to mind from the list below?

☐ Someone who makes me feel good about myself

☐ Someone who is interested in my opinion

☐ Someone who tells me how well I am doing

☐ Someone I can talk to if I am worried

☐ Someone who makes me stop and think about what I am doing

☐ Someone who makes me laugh and I can have fun with

☐ Someone who introduces me to new ideas, interests or new people

☐

☐

☐

☐

☐

The positive people on your list do not just have to be friends or family, colleagues or neighbours. The person you can talk to if you're worried, for example, could be a professional person that you see such as your GP, a counsellor or someone from an organization with a helpline. Maybe the person who introduces you to new ideas and interests could be the presenter of documentaries. Perhaps there's someone on the radio or TV who makes you laugh. The person who inspires you could be someone you've read about who's achieved something or who has overcome adversity in their life.

Looking for evidence

Looking for evidence for different ways of thinking can help you to see things in a more balanced way, and to consider both your negative and alternative thoughts as possibilities. Read the example below and then fill in your own 'negative/alternative thought record' on the following page. (There are also blank thought records at the back of the book.)

Situation:

My sister said she'd phone last night to discuss arrangements for a family party, but she didn't call.

Negative thought:

She's so unreliable. She's selfish and inconsiderate. She doesn't care about me.

How much do you believe this thought on a scale of 1-10?

10

What evidence do you have to support this thought?

It's always me that has to phone her. Yet if she wants me to babysit, she doesn't hesitate to call

Alternative thought:

Maybe she just forgot.

What evidence do you have to support this alternative view?

Getting her children to bed can be a struggle for her. Often they don't settle and get to sleep until quite late.

How much do you believe the alternative thought on a scale of 1-10?

7

Situation:

Negative thought:

How much do you believe this thought on a scale of 1-10?

What evidence do you have to support this thought?

Alternative thought:

What evidence do you have to support this alternative view?

How much do you believe the alternative thought on a scale of 1-10)?

How it works

Believing

How do I make myself believe the alternative thoughts?

You don't. Don't try and *make* yourself believe the alternative thoughts – just practise jotting down a few negative thoughts and the evidence 'for and against'. Your aim right now is simply to:

(1.) recognize that there **are** alternative ways of thinking

(2.) find evidence that can help support the alternative thoughts.

Keep it real

Alternative thoughts should be a more optimistic, though still realistic, alternative.

Make your alternative thoughts something that you can believe in. If your negative thought is 'I'd like to invite friends round for dinner but I'm not a good cook,' you're more likely to believe an alternative thought along the lines of 'I do have a couple of favourite recipes I do well,' rather than 'I'm actually a really good cook!'

Complete the realistic thought in the example below, then add your own examples.

Negative thought:

I'm going to totally fail this interview. They're going to think I'm wasting their time.

Unrealistic alternative thought:

I'm going to do really really well. They'll think I'm great and offer me the job.

Realistic thought?

Negative thought:

Unrealistic alternative thought:

Realistic thought?

Talk to yourself

When it comes to persuading yourself about something, research shows that in a variety of situations, if you address yourself by your own name, your chances of doing well can increase significantly.

It might seem weird, but it can focus your thinking and motivate you. Rather than telling yourself for example, 'I can do this' address yourself using your name: 'Amy, you can do this.' Try it!

Thought-changing prompts

When you notice that negative thoughts or images are starting to enter your mind, to prompt you to come up with alternative thoughts, try one of these;

- ☐ If you're sitting down, stand up.

- ☐ If you're standing up, sit down.

- ☐ If you're indoors go to a different room

- ☐ If you're outside, change the direction in which you're walking.

Alternatively, think of someone you've always found difficult to get on with (a family member, the friend of a friend, a neighbour or a colleague). Put aside your beliefs and opinions about them and see something new about them. Look for something positive. It could be an aspect of their personality, their attitude, something about the way they interact with others or something about how they work.

It takes but one positive thought when given a chance to survive and thrive to overpower an entire army of negative thoughts.

Dr. Robert H. Schuller

Remember

There are three main types of challenging questions you can ask yourself:

o Questions about how helpful your thinking is: whether your thoughts make you feel good or bad and do or don't get you what you want.

o Questions about the reality of your thinking: how much of what you think could happen is real, definite and true rather than just possible.

o Questions about alternative explanations: other ways of interpreting and explaining things.

Questions about how helpful your thoughts are:

o In what way is it helpful for me to think like this?

Questions about reality:

o What is the evidence for the negative thoughts – what did I think would happen?

o What is the evidence for an alternative thought – how certain am I on a scale of 1–10?

Questions about alternative explanations:

o How would a friend perceive this? What would they say to me?

o If the situation was reversed what positive things would I say to a friend if they were the one thinking negatively about this?

Let it go

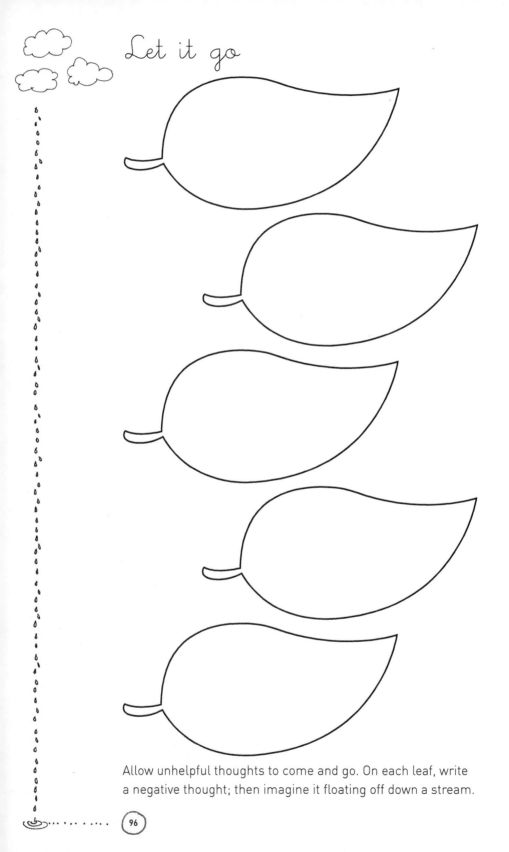

Allow unhelpful thoughts to come and go. On each leaf, write a negative thought; then imagine it floating off down a stream.

We are what we repeatedly do. Excellence then, is not an act, but a habit.

Aristotle

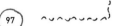

How it works

Developing good habits

Am I going to have to write down my thoughts, alternative thoughts, evidence etc. forever?

If you are serious about wanting to change things for the better, you will need to fill in quite a lot of negative/alternative thought records. (There is a blank template at the back of the book for you to copy.) You're not going to have to do this forever.

What you're aiming for is to get into the habit of noticing when your thoughts and responses are negative, then challenging your thoughts and looking for more helpful, positive ways of thinking. This will gradually become easier until you can do it in your head automatically, and it becomes your new, good habit.

You're not always going to notice your negative thoughts at the time they're happening. What you can do though, is find time during each day to think back and recall any instances in the day that you were thinking or behaving negatively.

Can't I just do all this in my head?

Writing out your thoughts is more powerful for a number of reasons:

o It helps you to empty your mind – to get those thoughts out of your head and onto paper or a screen. You're 'externalizing' your thoughts by writing them down.

o 'Seeing' your thoughts helps to give you a more objective perspective.

o You're more likely to notice regularly reoccurring patterns of thinking and the beliefs that support them

o Writing out negative/alternative thought records provide a record of progress.

Regularly writing out negative/alternative thought records helps train your brain get into a good habit so that eventually it will become second nature for you to dispute your thoughts and to think of more helpful alternative thoughts. Eventually you'll get to a point where you've trained your brain to simply think in positive, helpful ways.

As with establishing any habit, the more you do it, the sooner it will become automatic.

Do I need to wait for a drama or crisis?

No! Feeling irritated because you forgot to drink your coffee and now it's cold is just as valid a thought to note down and evaluate as those that accompany bigger worrries, such as about redundancy or a relationship break-up. The thought itself doesn't have to be momentous – write it down.

If ... then ...

You can help make writing negative/alternative thought records a habit by creating links that connect a new habit to an already established habit. For example, you might be in the habit of sitting down with a cup of tea when you come home from work each day. You could choose to link the activity of writing negative/alternative thought records with the habit of drinking a cup of tea.

By attaching a new habit (writing a negative/alternative thought record) to an already established habit (when you arrive home each day and have a cup of tea), you are using the 'If ... then...' technique: *If* you're having a cup of tea when you get home, *then* you'll write a negative/alternative thought record.

You can use this technique in other areas of your life. For example, if you want to get into the habit of more exercise:

*If I need to go up a couple floors at work, **then** I won't take the lift, I'll walk up the stairs.*

*If I'm taking the bus or tube, **then** I'll get off one stop earlier.*

*If I'm using the car, **then** I'll park my car ten minutes from my destination and walk the rest of the way.*

Complete the sentences below, then add your own 'If …
then …' sentences.

If I'm.. then
    I could sort out the recycling.

If I'm.. then
    I could clean out the fridge.

If I'm.. then
    I could change the sheets and duvet cover.

If I'm.. then
    I could clean the loo.

If I'm..then I
    could drink a glass of water.

If..

then...

If..

then...

If..

then...

If..

then...

If..

then...

What's in a word?

Won't, will, can't, can

Small, simple changes to the words you use can make a big difference to the way you think; they can really help you think and behave in helpful, positive ways.

Instead of saying, 'I *won't* get there for another hour', a more positive way of saying this would be simply, 'I *will* get there in an hour'.

Instead of 'I won't know until tomorrow', leave out the word 'won't' and say instead 'I will know tomorrow'.

What do you think is an alternative to this sentence?

I can't do it until next week.

Alternative sentence:

'Never ever' and 'always'

Words like 'always' and 'never' are often misused because the statements that include them are rarely true. For instance, 'I always forget things' is probably not true. You don't *always* forget things really, do you? It would far more realistic to say 'I *often* forget things' or 'I *sometimes* forget things.'

Be more aware of the words you use. It's okay to pause and organize your thoughts so that you can phrase your thoughts – and what you say out loud – in a positive way. And if you catch yourself using negative words and phrases mid-sentence, stop and rephrase what you want to say in more positive terms.

The power of 'but'

A useful way to change negative, unhelpful thoughts into more helpful thoughts is to follow the negative thought with a 'but' and then complete the sentence:

I don't think I can do this, but I'll try and if it looks like I can't manage, I'll ask for help.'

I'm so unfit, but I can exercise and get fitter.

These sentences started out as negative thoughts. Complete each sentence below to turn it into a positive thought.

I'm so nervous about meeting these people, but ...

I've let my friend down by cancelling our night out together, but ...

I didn't get the job, but ...

It's not fair; all my friends have better jobs than me, but ...

I don't like living here, but ...

The word 'but' encourages you to complete your sentence with something positive.

If you could just add a 'but' to every negative thought you produced, you could transform all negative thoughts into positive ones!

What's a negative thought you've had that you can turn into a positive one with the simple use of a 'but'?

I ...

but ...

Anytime you catch yourself saying a negative sentence, add the word 'but'. This prompts you to follow up with a positive sentence.

'And' not 'but'

How often do your thoughts start positively but end negatively?

Look at these two sentences:

I went for a run, but I only managed to get round the park twice.

It's nice of them to invite me to dinner, but it was probably because someone else dropped out.

'But' is a minimizing word that devalues the positive thought before it. Replacing the word 'but' with 'and' creates a much more positive meaning. By using the word 'and' you make it more likely that you will also come up with a solution. 'But' is final. 'And' implies there's still more to come, as you can read here.

I went for a run and I managed to get round the park twice and tomorrow I'm going to try and do three times.

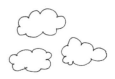

It's nice of them to invite me to dinner and I'm looking forward to it.

Each time, the word 'and' compels you to complete the sentence in a positive way.

Look back at page 59 'Thoughts about your goals'. This time, write out a goal and replace the word 'but' with 'and' and then finish the sentence.

Goal:

Thought:

and

Goal:

Thought:

and

Goal:

Thought:

and

Listen to other people

You can learn a lot about the effect of the language we all use just by listening to other people. Listen to the people around you and to people talking on TV and radio. Listen out for negative words and phrases and try to think of positive alternatives.

Watch a half-hour soap opera on TV or listen to one on the radio. Write down each time a negative word or sentence is used. Then write down a more positive word or sentence.

Negative word or sentence:

Alternative word or sentence:

The thinking friend and the thinking foe

Separate your thoughts from yourself by assigning characters to be the bearers of your thoughts. Imagine that you have two characters – cartoon characters – one sitting on your right shoulder and the other on your left shoulder.

On the right-hand side sits a character that's open minded, supportive and helpful. For example, Baloo the bear (*The Jungle Book*) or Lisa (*The Simpsons*).

On the left-hand side sits a character that's negative, blaming critical and miserable. For example, Ursula (*The Little Mermaid*) or Scar (*The Lion King*).

Choose characters that resonate with you. They don't have to be cartoon characters. They can be actors, music or sports stars, characters from movies and TV that you admire or dislike.

When something happens that makes you aware of your thoughts, listen and see which side is telling you this. Is it the supporter or the opposer?

If the thought is negative and unhelpful, ask the thinking foe some challenging questions. Listen to what the foe says and continue challenging. Your thinking friend can chime in any time as well.

When the thinking friend character gives you a helpful thought, touch your right shoulder and thank your supporter.

Throw-away thoughts

Throw your thoughts away. Once you have an alternative thought that you can believe, write down the negative thought on a piece of paper, then tear it up or screw it up and throw it in the bin.

Alternatively, text it to yourself, or write it on your computer, then press 'delete'.

Remember

o Rather than spend time and energy trying to *stop* negative thoughts, CBT encourages you to *change* your thoughts.

o Challenging your negative thoughts interrupts them and stops them from snowballing. This frees you to start thinking and responding in more positive ways. Recognizing that the way you're thinking isn't helpful – that it doesn't make you feel good or help you to get what you want – can prompt you to look at things differently.

o Your mind has a tendency to, first and foremost, notice and pay attention to experiences that match pre-existing thoughts and beliefs. Evidence to support an alternative view can often be outside of your awareness so you need to search hard for it.

o Looking for evidence for different ways of thinking can help you to see things in a more balanced way, and to consider both your negative and alternative thoughts as possibilities.

o Make your alternative thoughts something that you can believe in: a more optimistic, though still realistic, alternative.

o Regularly writing out thought records helps train your brain to get into a good habit so that eventually it will become second nature for you to dispute your thoughts and to think of more helpful alternatives. Eventually you'll get to a point where you've trained your brain to automatically think in positive helpful ways.

o Be more aware of the words you use. Small, simple changes to the words you use can make a big difference to the way you think; they can really help you think and behave in helpful, positive ways.

o It's okay to pause and organize your thoughts so that you can phrase them – and what you say out loud – in a positive way. And if you catch yourself using negative words and phrases mid-sentence, stop and rephrase what you want to say in more positive terms.

Chapter 4

Thoughts and physical feelings

Lemon meditation

Imagine a bright yellow lemon in your hand. Notice how it feels to your touch. The skin is both smooth and bumpy. Smell the lemon – its unique, fresh, lemon smell. Now imagine cutting the lemon in half; picture the edge of the knife breaking the skin, releasing a fine, lemon mist.

Now take one half of the lemon and cut a slice. Again, smell the lemon; the sharp, fresh citrus scent. Touch the lemon to your lips.

Is your mouth watering as if you've actually tasted the lemon? This just goes to show how thoughts can create a physical response. It shows the power of the mind to create a physical reaction in our bodies.

Thoughts and feelings

Think of a situation recently where things didn't go well for you. Perhaps a friend let you down, you made a mistake at work, you had a dispute on the phone with a service provider or someone said something that left you feeling humiliated. Write down what you can recall of the thoughts you had about this at the time. How did you feel physically? For example:

Situation:

Made a mistake at work.

Thought:

What an idiot. I'm hopeless. Everyone is going to think I can't cope. I'm going to get into trouble about this.

Physical feeling:

Stomach in knots. Tightness in my throat.

Situation:

Thought:

Physical feeling (circle the area or areas where you felt it):

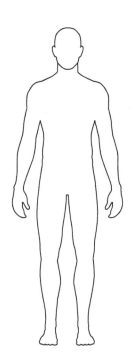

Now recall a situation that was a happy one. Perhaps you achieved something you had been working towards, or someone paid you a compliment or did something really nice for you. Write down what happened and your thoughts about this situation as you can recall them.

How did these thoughts make you feel? How did you feel physically? For example:

Situation:

Offered a job/place on a course
I really wanted.

Thought:

Brilliant! I'm so pleased.

Physical feeling:

Light and bouncy!

Situation:

Thought:

Physical feeling (circle the area or areas where you felt it:

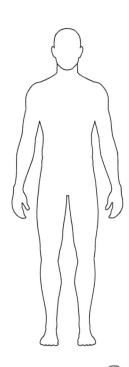

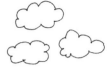

Emotions have a physical aspect – stomach churning, tenseness, fidgeting, trembling etc. Often, you might notice more how you're physically feeling than what you're thinking; physical feelings can alert you to notice what you're thinking.

Circle where you feel happiness and love. Put crosses where you feel frustration, sadness, disappointment, anxiety and uncertainty.

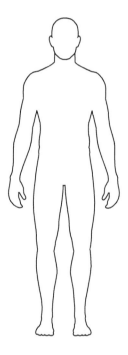

The physical symptoms of anger and excitement are often the same – heart thumping, rapid breathing, tenseness, trembling. What makes the two different? Your thoughts and your behaviour.

Melting ice cube meditation

Place an ice cube on the palm of your hand. Feel the texture of the ice. Watch the ice melt and the water drip through your fingers.

What are your thoughts and feelings?

The ice cube meditation can help you recognize the impermanence of mental and physical discomfort and your emotional response to it.

Chapter 5
Beliefs

True or false?

Put a tick next to those facts you believe to be true and a cross next to the ones you believe to be false.

(1.)   The Great Wall of China is visible from space.   ☐

(2.)   Bats are blind.   ☐

(3.)   Goldfish have a memory of only five seconds.   ☐

(4.)   Pure white cats with blue eyes are more likely to be deaf.   ☐

(5.)   Three wise men came to visit Jesus when he was born.   ☐

(6.)   Caffeine dehydrates you.   ☐

(7.)   We only use 10 per cent of our brains.   ☐

(8.)   Hair and fingernails continue growing after you die.   ☐

(9.)   A shot of whisky or brandy will warm you up.   ☐

(10.) It takes 21 days to change a habit.   ☐

Are you certain about your answers? How can you be 100 per cent sure? What evidence do you have for each statement you have decided is true or false? Google the answers. Go on – make the effort to find out if your assumptions are correct.

(Answers at the back of the book.)

Personal beliefs

Tick which of these statements you think are true. Then add your own beliefs about yourself, other people or the way the world works.

☐ I should know what I want from life by now.

☐ Other people's approval is important.

☐ With everything I do, unless it's perfect, it won't be good enough.

☐ Difficult patches in life are temporary.

☐ You can't please all the people all the time.

☐ I can't change – it's too late.

☐ For one reason or another, at some point, people are always going to leave me.

☐ I can't do things on my own.

☐ Others should show respect and appreciation when you do something for them.

☐ Life is unfair.

☐ As long as you try your best that's all that matters.

☐ I'm weak.

☐ I don't deserve success or happiness.

☐ It's never too late to learn.

☐ I always seem to do the wrong thing.

☐ Things never work out for me, no matter what I do.

☐ I'm not clever

☐

☐

☐

Which of your beliefs are positive and helpful and which ones are limiting and unhelpful?

How it works

Beliefs

I'm still finding it hard to believe alternative thoughts. Why is that?

If you find it difficult to believe alternative thoughts it's helpful to look at the beliefs and assumptions that lie beneath your thoughts.

For example, your thought might be, 'I'm upset because my friend showed up late for lunch. She doesn't really care about me.' The underlying belief could be, 'I'm not a likeable person'. If you firmly believe yourself to be an unlikeable person then you'll need to work on changing that belief in order to consider more helpful, positive thoughts about your likeability.

Where do our beliefs about ourselves, other people and the world come from?

Whatever your beliefs, you certainly weren't born with them. Many of your beliefs and patterns of thinking have developed over the years as a result of your upbringing – the influences of your family and friends, your environment, education, media, culture and so on. As children, we usually accept the beliefs and ways of thinking of other people.

Even if this produces thoughts, feelings and behaviours that are limiting and self-defeating, we suppress the instinct to question our own thinking.

So all my beliefs come from my childhood?

Not all of them. Beliefs can also develop from events that have happened to you as an an adult. They can be strengthened in adulthood; your beliefs can be further confirmed by 'proof'. For example, if you failed to get a job promotion you applied for it could confirm your 'I'm never good enough' belief.

What's the difference between thoughts and beliefs?

Thoughts tend to be about specific events. Beliefs are generalizations – they're principles and conclusions you come to based on only a few examples of an experience or situation. Like thoughts, beliefs leave you feeling sure about the truth of something even if you don't have firm evidence. Your negative beliefs generate your negative unhelpful thoughts. Your positive beliefs generate your positive thoughts.

Can I do anything about my unhelpful beliefs?

Yes! You don't have to stick with these limiting beliefs! Beliefs are like a wet swimming costume – they can be difficult to peel off; a struggle, but not impossible.

Remember

o As previously mentioned, you have a system in your brain called the 'reticular activating system' (RAS) The RAS filters out everything that doesn't fit with your core beliefs. So, your mind has a tendency to stick with thoughts that correspond with your core beliefs.

o You can though, change your beliefs. Then, your brain will be more aware of events and interpretations that fit with the new beliefs.

Uncovering your beliefs

Limiting beliefs are often unconscious and unquestioned, which makes them hard to find. There is, though, a simple way to help identify your limiting beliefs: use the word 'because'.

When 'because' appears in a sentence it's followed by a reason; an explanation of a belief: 'I can't change jobs... because... I am too old.'

'Because' can help you uncover your beliefs.

Write down a problem or difficulty you have, or something that you want to happen – an issue at work, with friends, family etc. -followed by the word 'because'. Then complete the sentence with as many reasons as come to your mind.

Issue:

Reason:

Reason:

Reason:

Reason:

Give each 'reason' a score from 1–10 (1 = a slight possibility; 10 = definitely true).

Now you have identified 'reasons', you have identified some limiting beliefs. The one with the highest score is your main limiting belief.

Rules for living

Your beliefs create assumptions which are your 'rules for living'. We all have rules for living.

Helpful belief:

Difficult patches in life are temporary.

Rule for living:

Be patient; things **will** get better.

Unhelpful belief:

I can never be good enough.

Rule for living:

Don't do anything that might be beyond my ability. It'll save me the pain of rejection.

Write down a few of your own and then see if you can identify any rules that might have come from your beliefs.

Belief:

Rule for living:

Belief:

Rule for living:

Belief:

Rule for living:

Your beliefs pave your way to success or they block you.

Marsha Sineta

Challenging your beliefs

You can adjust your beliefs in the same way you adjust thoughts – by weakening old beliefs and identifying and strengthening new, more helpful beliefs.

Ask yourself what *advantages* there are in hanging on to your old beliefs. How do you benefit from these beliefs? What do you gain? Then ask yourself what the *disadvantages* of continuing to hold such beliefs are. What do you stand to lose and miss out on?

Belief:

Advantages and benefits to believing this:

Disadvantages of believing this:

Belief:

Advantages and benefits to believing this:

Disadvantages of believing this:

Creating more helpful, optimistic beliefs

Write the negative beliefs you've identified in the first column. In the second column write down more balanced alternative beliefs.

Belief:	Alternative belief:
I'm unlikeable	I've got one or two qualities that people like

Evidence for beliefs

Identify evidence you have to support a belief. Then look for evidence that could support an alternative belief.

Belief:

If things go wrong, I always think that I'm the one responsible for putting things right.

How strongly I believe this:

100%

Alternative, more helpful belief:

It can't be *all* my fault. I don't have to make their situation my own.

How strongly I believe this:

20%

Evidence to support my new belief:

Other people are often involved in the things that go wrong.

Further evidence, whenever it appears, to support the new belief:

I'm not the one who let them down. I'm not responsible for their disappointment.

How strongly I now believe this:

60%

Belief:

How strongly I believe this:

Alternative, more helpful belief:

How strongly I believe this:

Evidence to support my new belief:

Further evidence, whenever it appears, to support the new belief:

How strongly I believe this:

As you add further evidence for your new beliefs, check your belief rating. Don't expect to reach 100 per cent. Simply an 'on balance' view will be a good result and enable you to view situations in a more realistic way. You are simply training your mind to become more open to the possibility that you are being too hard on yourself or others and that a more balanced view helps you to feel better.

You are not trying to make yourself believe that something is true or not, you are simply considering what the most open, helpful belief is.

Remember

o Talk to yourself. If you address yourself by your own name, you increase your ability to believe the alternative belief. Rather than telling yourself, for example, 'You can do things on your own' address yourself using your name: 'Louise, you can do things on your own'.

o Self-talk can be positive: kind, encouraging and empowering.

Change your beliefs and you'll change your thoughts.

Change your thoughts and you'll change your habits.

Change your habits and your life opens to unlimited possibility.

Gail Lynne Goodwin

Shoulda, coulda, musta

Whenever you have a thought or say the words 'should', 'must' and 'ought' in a sentence, you imply that you have a duty; there's an absolute requirement that you or someone else *has* to do or is expected to do something. On the other hand, the word 'could' tells you that you're making a choice about what to think and do or not think and do.

Write down three sentences using 'should', 'must' or 'ought' in a way that relates to negative thoughts that you have/had about yourself. Then write the sentences again, having binned the 'shoulds', 'musts' and 'oughts'.

I *should* know what I want from life
I *could* know what I want from life

I should

I could

I must always

I could

I ought to

I could

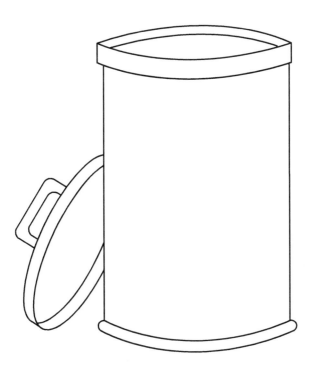

Write the words 'should', 'shouldn't', 'must', 'mustn't', 'ought' and 'ought not' inside the rubbish bin.

Star breathing meditation

Trace the outline of the star with your finger. Start at any 'breathe in' side, hold your breath at the point, then breathe out. Keep going until you've gone around the whole star.

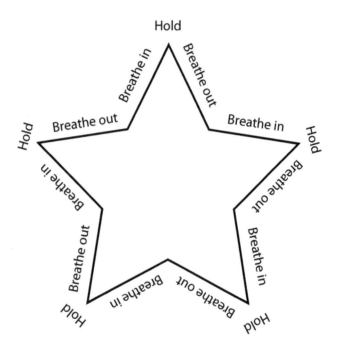

Remember

- Negative, unhelpful thoughts are not always so easy to challenge and dismiss. This can be because of the beliefs and assumptions that lie beneath your thoughts. You don't have to stick with these limiting beliefs!

- Ask yourself what *advantages* there are in hanging on to your old beliefs. How do you benefit from these beliefs? What do you gain? Then ask yourself what the *disadvantages* of continuing to hold such beliefs are. What do you stand to lose and miss out on?

- Identify evidence you have to support a belief. Then look for evidence that could support an alternative belief.

- As you add further evidence for your new beliefs, check your belief rating. Don't expect to reach 100 per cent. You are not trying to make yourself believe that something is true or not, you are simply considering what the most open, helpful belief is.

- Whenever you have a thought or say the words 'should', 'must' and 'ought' in a sentence, you imply that you have a duty; there's an absolute requirement that you or someone else *has* to do or is expected to do something. On the other hand, the word 'could' tells you that you're making a choice about what to think and do or not think and do.

Chapter 6
Behaviour

Remember

- What you think influences what you do and don't do.
- It's also true that what you do influences what you think. Just as, in any one situation, there is more than one way to think, there is also more than one way to respond and behave.

Avoidance

Are there any situations you often avoid? Tick any of the examples below then add your own.

☐ You get invited to a party. You're anxious about having to make small talk, thinking 'I won't know what to say. People will think I'm boring or stupid'. You make an excuse and don't go.

☐ You have to drive or take a bus or train journey somewhere you've not been to before. You think 'I'll get lost. I'll panic and not know what to do'. You decide not to go.

☐ You want to talk to someone about their difficult behaviour. You think, 'They won't like it; they'll get defensive and we'll have a row'. You choose not to say anything.

☐ You have to cancel going to the cinema with a friend at short notice. You think 'I feel bad for having let her down, she was looking forward to this' and you avoid seeing her for a while, hoping she'll forget about it.

☐ You've signed up for a class in a subject that you're keen to learn. You get to the college and think 'I can't face walking into a room full of strangers' and you turn around and go home.

☐ Your elderly aunt has been in a care home for six months now. You keep meaning to visit but still haven't got round to it. You think 'I've left it so long, it'd be embarrassing to visit now'. You don't visit.

☐ Your home is becoming cluttered; you have things you no longer want or need. You keep meaning to sort through everything and have a clearout but you think 'There's too much stuff. I don't know where to start. I'll leave it for another time'.

☐

☐

☐

☐

☐

☐

Steering clear of potentially stressful situations is known as 'avoidance behaviour'. If total avoidance is not possible, you may resort to 'escape behaviour'; leaving or escaping a situation as soon as you can.

Avoidance and escape behaviours – also known as 'safety behaviours' – may make you feel better in the short term, but in the long term, you don't learn how to cope with your fears and take control of situations.

Energy spent on avoidance and escape could be better spent on thinking about you can do – not what you think you can't do.

Case study

As Ashley grew up she was often told by her parents that she 'could do better'. This gave Ashley an 'I'm not good enough' belief.

Although she is good at her job, every time an opportunity for promotion comes up Ashley shies away from it. Her thoughts are, 'I'd like a new role but I'd only mess up and then I'd be out of a job completely. Best to stay where I am.'

Ashley's view is that if you don't try then you can't fail. Better to do nothing at all than to do something that doesn't work out well is how Ashley copes with most aspects of her life.

Although Ashley wants a partner, she thinks it better to turn down a date than accept it and the other person not call her again. And although she loves singing, better not to accept the invitation to join the choir in case they see she isn't the world's best singer.

While this way of thinking and behaving keep Ashley 'safe' it also strengthens her 'I'm not good enough at anything' belief.

Avoidance works very well for Ashley. But it maintains her problems. Ashley's actions (or inactions) simply confirm her view of herself as someone who is never good enough. Ashley never discovers that she could handle a job promotion or that accepting an invitation might be the first step in finding a partner or a fulfilling interest. By risking nothing – by staying in her comfort zone – Ashley is trapped in her limited life which in turn reinforces her 'I'm not good enough for better' views.

If you're like Ashley and you avoid challenges, you don't learn how to cope with your fears and take control of situations. You don't give yourself the chance to discover what you could actually be capable of and you don't give yourself the opportunity to feel good about yourself for having achieved something.

It doesn't have to be this way!

Life begins at the end of your comfort zone.

Neale Donald Walsh

How it works

Stepping out of your comfort zone

What's a comfort zone?

When you're in your comfort zone you only do things in ways that you are comfortable with, within certain limits. For example going to a restaurant with friends could be your comfort zone. Going to a restaurant on your own could be out of your comfort zone. It could even take you into a panic zone!

Why should I leave my comfort zone?

Take a small step outside your comfort zone and each time you do, you widen your thoughts and beliefs about what you're capable of doing.

Where am I going if I step outside my comfort zone?

You'll be stepping into the confidence-building zone (also known as the courage zone).

What do I need to do?

Choose a situation and do something slightly different and challenging – something that's just one small step away from what you're normally comfortable with. (CBT calls this process 'graded exposure'.)

How I can be sure that anything I do differently will be helpful?

You can't be sure. But what you can do is reflect on each change of behaviour and learn from it. If the first step you take outside your comfort zone is successful, you then take another step. If it doesn't work out, you simply identify what would be a smaller step to take in that situation. And then take that easier step.

In any one situation, if you push yourself too hard and too far out of your comfort zone you can find yourself in a panic zone; overwhelmed by anxiety and stress. But step *just outside* your comfort zone into the 'confidence-building zone' and, although you'll feel challenged, you are more likely to achieve things in a controlled, managed way; you won't feel so stressed that you retreat back into your comfort zone.

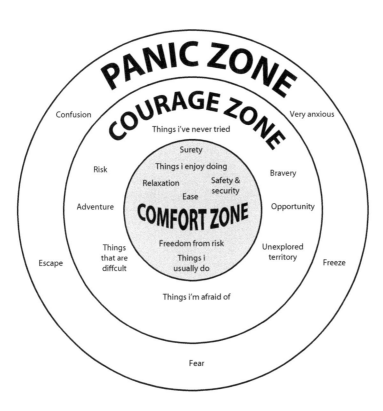

Leaving your comfort zone: for and against

Think of something you would like to be able to do, have or be but don't because you think you'll fail. Put a tick next to your reasons for and against stepping outside your comfort zone. Add your own reasons too.

For

- ☐ I'll stretch myself
- ☐ I can be courageous
- ☐ It'll build my confidence
- ☐ It'll open up new opportunities and experiences
- ☐ I'll see more. Do more.
- ☐ I'll learn new things about myself; what I'm really capable of
- ☐ I'll discover good things about other people and the world
- ☐ I'll feel a sense of achievement
- ☐
- ☐

Against

- ☐ Everything is fine as it is
- ☐ It's scary
- ☐ It takes persistent repeated effort
- ☐ It's risky; it might not work out
- ☐ I might end up taking one step forward and two steps back
- ☐
- ☐

Which reasons are most helpful for you – the reasons 'for' or 'against'?

Writing out the steps

Choose a situation – a problem or difficulty you'd like to overcome, or something you'd like the confidence to do but, for one reason or another, you don't think you'd be able to do it. Think about what you would like to be able to do. This is your goal.

Think about what aspect of that situation you *do* feel comfortable with and capable of doing. This is your starting point. Then think of something you can do – one small step you can take that will enable you to achieve and feel good about. Next, make a list of small steps you could take.

Don't just 'give things a go' – write out first every step you plan to take.

Goal:

Step 1:

Step 2:

Step 3:

Step 4:

Step 5:

Step 6:

Step 7:

Step 8:

Graded exposure

CBT calls the step-by-step process 'graded exposure'. Exposure involves gradually doing the thing that you find stressful until you feel comfortable with each step.

1. **Joel wants to declutter his kitchen but the thought of sorting, tidying and throwing out all the crockery, pans, equipment, cutlery and utensils is overwhelming him. Currently, he feels comfortable throwing out broken equipment, cracked or chipped crockery. His goal is to only keep the things he regularly uses.**

Joel's written a list of small steps he could take. He plans to take one step every day for a week. Put them in order of least scary to most difficult.

☐ Take unwanted items to charity shop.

☐ Choose one drawer or cupboard to sort out.

☐ Repeat the process with another drawer or cupboard on another day.

☐ Take out everything from the chosen drawer or cupboard and put onto the table.

☐ Take out broken, chipped or cracked things and put in a box.

☐ Put back in the cupboard / drawer those items – crockery, pans, cutlery etc. – that I use often.

☐ Put unwanted items into a box.

(Answers at the back of the book.)

2. Sam would like to start an art class. He signed up for a class last term but when he got to the college he couldn't face walking into a room full of strangers so he went home.

Sam's written a list of small steps he could take. Sam plans to take one step every day for a week. Put them in order of least scary to most difficult.

☐ Go to the first class – be the first to arrive.

☐ Before the course begins, go to the college on a busy day on my own and have a coffee in the cafe.

☐ Go to the open day and meet the tutor in the room where the class will take place.

☐ Before the course begins, go to the college with a friend and have a coffee in the café.

☐ Phone a friend for encouragement on my way to the first class.

(Answers at the back of the book.)

A behavioural experiment

Use this page to carry out a 'behavioural experiment'.

Goal:

Comfort zone (what I feel comfortable doing)

First step out of my comfort zone:

How do I feel about doing it? On a scale of 1-10
how strong is that feeling?

What actually happened?

How do I feel about doing it again? On a scale of
1-10 how strong is that feeling?

What have I learnt from this?

Next realistic, doable step:

How do I feel about doing it? On a scale of 1-10 how strong is that feeling?

What actually happened?

How do I feel about doing it again? On a scale of 1-10 how strong is that feeling?

What have I learned from this?

Next realistic, doable step:

How do I feel about doing it? On a scale of 1-10 how strong is that feeling?

What actually happened?

How do I feel about doing it again? On a scale of 1-10 how strong is that feeling?

What have I learned from this?

How it works
The learning cycle

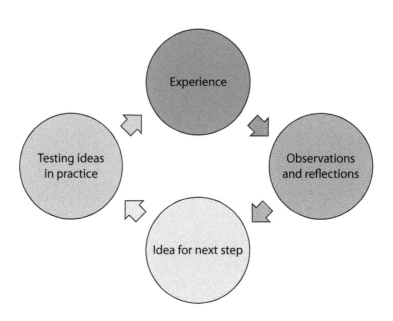

To fully learn something – for it to really mean something to you and to become a good habit – involves a cycle of doing and thinking.

How do you eat an elephant? One bite at a time.

Anon

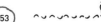

Remember

- Every time you do something or avoid doing something in a way that corresponds with your negative thoughts, you strengthen the idea that your thoughts are true, logical and rational.

- It works both ways: every time you do something that goes well, you're more likely to have positive thoughts about the situation, to believe those positive helpful thoughts and to see them as true, logical and rational.

Be brave. Take risks. Nothing can substitute experience.

Paulo Coelho

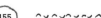

How it works

Experimenting and learning

Stepping out of my comfort zone by 'experimenting' seems to take the pressure off - is that the idea?

Yes! Each time you prepare to step out of your comfort zone, think of it as carrying out an experiment; you're trying out new ways of behaving and seeing what happens. Just like a scientist setting up an experiment for the purpose of discovering something unknown, you just take each step with no expectations other than to see what happens.

So with each 'experiment' - each step - I'm just focusing on doing it, seeing what happens and learning from it?

Again, yes! When the focus is on learning and improving, you're more likely to be calmer than if you thought you *had* to get it right.

An example of this is the difference between driving lessons and a driving test. When you're having a driving lesson you're simply focused on learning and improving. But typically, when you take your test, the pressure is on; you're worrying about your driving and trying to avoid mistakes. The pressure to do well and avoid mistakes can just make you stressed and anxious and more likely to not do well.

Doing things one step at a time gives you time to look at what is working and what isn't, and to decide if you need to change tactics. So, as you go through each step, review the outcome. What's worked? What helped and went well?

Just imagine

Keep your mind focused on one step at a time. Tell yourself, 'This is what I'm going to do next' and then just focus on that one step you're taking.

It's important to visualize each and every step. Create images for yourself where you see yourself coping and achieving successful outcomes. Instead of playing out the worst scenario in your mind, play out the best.

The more you imagine yourself coping and coming out the other side, the more likely it is to happen.

Remember

- What could feel impossible in one big leap, becomes a lot more doable as a series of smaller steps.

- It's something you've done many times before. Any task, activity or goal, anything you've achieved – from getting up and going to work to moving house – has been the result of a series of steps.

- If you find that a step feels too difficult then break it up into something more manageable. Once you're comfortable with it you can take another step, and another, towards your final goal. Think in terms of pushing yourself just a little beyond your comfort zone.

- The aim is to strengthen your thoughts and beliefs that you *can* do things. Taking a step-by-step approach means you set yourself up for constant successes by achieving small targets along the way. You help yourself believe that you can do things because each step strengthens your beliefs about what you are capable of and encourages you to believe you can do a bit more with each step.

Minimizing risks

Still teetering on the edge? Finding it difficult to take the plunge? What's the worst that can happen? For each step write down what's the worst that could happen. Then think how you would deal with it.

Step:

Go to a cafe on my own.

Worst-case scenario:

I'll feel awkward and conspicuous.

How I could deal with that:

Take something to read.

Step:

Worst-case scenario:

How I could deal with that:

Test out a superstition

Do you believe that putting shoes on the table or putting an umbrella up indoors is unlucky? Test it. Put your shoes on the table. Open an umbrella indoors.

Do you think that if something bad or difficult *did* later happen it was *because* of the shoes or umbrella? Or because of your confirmation bias: because you looked for something to blame your 'bad luck' on?

Having courage

So often, avoiding fears can make them stronger and scarier; you can spend more time and energy avoiding what you fear than facing your fears and dealing with them. You need courage!

Courage means doing something *despite* your fearful thoughts.

Courage means accepting your fears then working out a series of steps to work past your fears and achieve your goal.

Think of something you'd like to do but you're worried it won't turn out well.

Courage gives you the ability to do something despite fear, doubt and lack of confidence. There is power in doing. You have to start with courage; that first step is usually a courageous one.

You gain strength, courage, and confidence by every
experience in which you really stop to look fear in the face.

Eleanor Roosevelt

Courage is a habit, a virtue. You get it by courageous acts.
It's like you learn to swim by swimming. You learn courage
by couraging.

Brene Brown

Good habit

Courage boosting

Get into the habit of being courageous:

- Remind yourself *why* you're going to do something – this can give you the motivation and courage you need to take the necessary first step. Focusing on why you're doing something and what you want to achieve, and keeping that in your mind, stops you from allowing feelings of doubt, uncertainty and fear to creep in. Focus on the benefits, not the difficulties. Instead of thinking about how hard something is, think about what you'll get out of it. Focus on how good you'll feel when you've done it.

- Don't overthink it. The more you think about whether you should or shouldn't do something the less likely you are to take that first courageous step. Courage can be prone to leaking so the longer you wait, the less of it you'll have. Once you've decided to do something, don't wait, do it!

- Rather than fight feelings of fear and doubt, acknowledge and accept them. Tell yourself 'I'm feeling scared. I'm not sure about this.' Then push past those thoughts and feelings and tell yourself 'But I can do this.' Feel the fear. And then do it.

- Take a deep breath then hold it. The space created by pausing gives you long enough to engage your courage. The second you breathe out, use that moment you have created for yourself to make the leap and take that first step.

- Picture everything going well. Imagine that everything will work out. Visualize it.

- Be inspired by courageous people. When you're trying to stretch yourself beyond your apparent limits, there's a part of you that wonders whether it can actually be done. A courageous role model is a constant reminder that the answer is 'yes'. Who's your role model for courage?

If you don't like something, change it; if you can't change it, change the way you think about it.

Mary Engelbreit

Affirmations

An affirmation is the assertion that something is valid and true.

Here are some affirmations: rational, positive statements to replace the negative and irrational thoughts that take-over when you feel anxious, stressed, angry or face other overwhelming situations. They offer reassurance that you can make it through a difficult situation.

Choose affirmations below that are meaningful and believable for you. Write out your own. Put them into your phone.

When you need courage and confidence, read them – out loud if possible – and repeat them until you start to feel better. If one statement in particular helps calm you most, just continue to repeat it to yourself, like a mantra.

Breathe slowly and deeply as you read your statements.

→ One step at a time.
→ Stop. Breathe.
→ I can do this.
→ I'm going to focus on my breathing until I know what to do.
→ I can be anxious/angry/sad and still deal with this.
→ I'm going to face this problem situation the best that I can.
→ I have done this before, and I can do it again.
→ I don't need to rush, I can take things slowly.
→ I'm stronger than I think.
→ It's okay to feel this way, it's a normal reaction.
→ Thoughts are just thoughts. They are not necessarily true.
→ This is difficult and uncomfortable, but it is only temporary.
→ I can get through this.
→ Slow. Down.
→ I can learn from this.
→ When this is over, I'll be pleased that I did it.

Write down your affirmations

Write down affirmations – coping thoughts – that relate to a difficult or distressing situation you are experiencing or have experienced. Something you can tell yourself that will help you get through. Use one of the affirmations on page 165 or make up your own.

Situation:

Affirmation (positive coping statement):

Remember

o Unhelpful negative behaviour can reinforce negative views.

o The idea that changing what you do can really change what you think is a key principle of CBT.

Imagination meditation

Try one of the following imagination meditations:

o Use your imagination. Breathe in like you're smelling the scent of a flower. Breathe out like you're blowing bubbles.

o Imagine breathing out to the ends of the universe and breathing from there back into your body.

o Breathe colour – imagine the colour of the air filling not just your lungs but your entire body.

Good habit

Stretch yourself

Which of these things would take you out of your comfort zone? What could present enough of a challenge to put you in the stretch zone? Practise making yourself just a little bit uncomfortable.

Do one thing every day that pushes you out of your comfort zone and feel your courage and confidence grow.

Here are some ideas:

- ☐ Get up or go to bed 30 minutes earlier.

- ☐ Change what you eat for breakfast.

- ☐ Take a different route to work, the supermarket, to visit friends and family, or on the school run.

- ☐ Get off the bus or tube one stop earlier and walk.

- ☐ Watch a programme or listen to music you wouldn't normally watch or listen to.

- ☐ Read a paper or magazine you'd never normally read.

- ☐ Use the stairs at work, not the lift.

- ☐ Look around a shop you wouldn't normally go into.

- ☐ Cook a new recipe for dinner.

Step outside

Look at your everyday routines and push yourself to do things a bit differently or a bit more. Write a list of five things you could do that would move you out of your comfort zone. Include things that won't involve too much of a stretch.

1. ___

2. ___

3. ___

4. ___

5. ___

What are your thoughts before you attempt these new routines?

1. ___

2. ___

3.
___

4.
___

5.
___

On a scale of 1–10, how easy was it? How comfortable did it make you feel? (10 = very easy and comfortable; 1 = difficult and uncomfortable). What are your thoughts afterwards?

1.
___

2.
___

3.
___

4.
___

5.
___

Get used to stepping outside your comfort zone. Make it a habit.

How it works

Making it a permanent habit

How long does it take to establish good habits?

Ten days? Three weeks? A couple of months? It's different for everyone – there are no hard and fast rules. There are four stages to changing from an unhelpful habit to a good, helpful habit:

1. At first, you are unaware of the possibility or need to change the way you think and behave. It's what you do.

2. At some point you move onto the next stage where you recognize and accept that you want things to change and you're open to possible solutions, ideas and advice. (Reading this book means that you're at this stage.) You know that it's not going to be easy but you intend to take steps to help you do something about it.

3. The next stage is the action stage, the stage when you actually make the changes. You try out new ways of thinking and behaving.

4. You maintain those changes and eventually a new habit is established – it becomes your new normal way of thinking or doing.

Is it that straightforward?

No. It's more of a cycle of change. You are likely to move through the cycle a number of times before permanently establishing more helpful ways of thinking and behaving.

So will I fall back to where I started?

No. Usually, you make progress and then slip back a few times until the new ways become your normal way of thinking and behaving. It's important that you remember this, so that if you do slip back to your old ways of thinking and behaving, you don't fall for the 'what the hell effect'.

What's the 'what the hell effect'?

It's when you slip back from a new habit you're working on. Then, you're far more likely to give up on the progress you've made. 'What the hell? I've blown it so I might as well forget about my good intentions.'

Minor setbacks and frustrating moments are habit killers; they give you an excuse to give up.

What to do?

Get things in perspective. For those 'what the hell moments', instead of giving up, think about and focus on what you have achieved in establishing your new good habit. Think positively! Know that you can always take up where you left off, tomorrow. Use a 'beginner's mind' approach.

What's beginner's mind?

'Beginner's mind' is a mindfulness concept. It encourages you to experience life in the present moment, to let go of mistakes – they're now in the past – and take a new perspective; to respond to things as if for the first time – as they are right now.

Which step?

Where are you today?

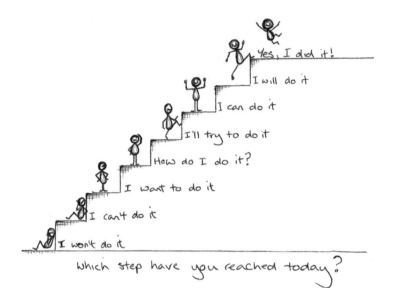

Yes, I did it!

I will do it

I can do it

I'll try to do it

How do I do it?

I want to do it

I can't do it

I won't do it

Which step have you reached today?

Be nice!

Kindness creates a positive mindset. When you look for opportunities to be kind you are making an effort to think in positive ways. It doesn't have to cost anything or take much time. You only need to be a bit more aware of other people to start seeing opportunities to be nice, considerate and kind.

Below are a few ideas. Add your own and check them off as you do them.

- ☐ Get in touch with someone you haven't been in contact with for a while. Write them a card, email or text just to let them know you were thinking about them.

- ☐ Notice the work someone does. It could be someone who serves you in a shop or café. Make a positive comment about their work or business.

- ☐ Send a surprise gift to a friend, for example a book from an online retailer. When you find something you know a friend would like, don't wait for a birthday or Christmas, send it now.

- ☐ Be friendly on public transport. Offer your seat on the train or bus to someone who you're aware needs it more that you.

- ☐ Did your colleague have a bad day today? Bring her a coffee tomorrow morning.

- ☐ Invite people out. Ask someone to do something nice with you – the cinema, a show, a walk, a meal.

- ☐ Say something nice on someone's Facebook or Twitter page, or on their blog or website. Don't just 'Like' something – make an effort to write a line or two of positive comments.

☐ Be polite on the road; be kind to other drivers. In a queue, let people in front of you.

☐ Hold the door open for someone and smile at them as you do so.

☐ Buy someone a coffee and cake or some fresh fruit – summer strawberries or raspberries. It could be your colleagues, a neighbour, a family member or friend. Whoever it is, surprise them.

☐

☐

☐

☐

Slip-ups

Finish this sentence:

If I fall into thinking or behaving in unhelpful ways, I can …

- a) Lose hope and give up
- b) Remind myself of what I've achieved so far and start again

Every day is a new beginning. Take a deep breath and start again.

Anon

Good habit

Three good things

At the end of each day write down three good things that have happened that day.

Even if you have a bad day, find three good things that happened. Maybe the sun was shining? You got an amusing text from a friend? You had something nice to eat? Just make an effort for a couple of weeks to identify the good things in your day. After a while, identifying and reflecting on small pleasures will become a habit. A good habit.

Day 1

Day 2

Day 3

Day 4

Day 5

Strengths and qualities

Tick each and every quality that applies to you.

☐ Adventurous	☐ Good natured	☐ Perceptive
☐ Adaptable	☐ Honest	☐ Practical
☐ Caring	☐ Helpful	☐ Precise
☐ Calm	☐ Hardworking	☐ Reassuring
☐ Co-operative	☐ Imaginative	☐ Reliable
☐ Curious	☐ Independent	☐ Resourceful
☐ Conscientious	☐ Innovative	☐ Resilient
☐ Courteous	☐ Logical	☐ Responsible
☐ Creative	☐ Loyal	☐ Realistic
☐ Dependable	☐ Intuitive	☐ Sense of humour
☐ Decisive	☐ Likeable	
☐ Diplomatic	☐ Meticulous	☐ Sincere
☐ Determined	☐ Methodical	☐ Sociable
☐ Empathic	☐ Observant	☐ Sympathetic
☐ Encouraging	☐ Optimistic	☐ Thorough
☐ Energetic	☐ Organized	☐ Tactful
☐ Fair	☐ Outgoing	☐ Tolerant
☐ Firm	☐ Persistent	☐ Tidy
☐ Flexible	☐ Patient	☐ Trustworthy
☐ Friendly	☐ Open minded	☐ Truthful
☐ Gentle	☐ Objective	☐ Understanding

Evidence again

Out of the strengths and qualities you ticked, choose your top five strengths and qualities.

Then, for each strength and quality, write a couple of sentences explaining how, when and why you've used that strength or quality.

Strength/Quality:

Evidence:

Strength/Quality:

Evidence:

Strength/Quality:

Evidence:

Strength/Quality:

Evidence:

Strength/Quality:

Evidence:

Live your life as if everything is rigged in your favour.

Arianna Huffington

Use your strengths

Think of something you want to be able to do. What strengths, skills and personal qualities do you already have that could contribute to developing your ability in that area?

Situation:

Strengths and qualities that could help me in that situation:

Make snap decisions

Look for opportunities to step outside your comfort zone.
Now and again, don't overthink it, just step straight out of
your comfort zone and do things differently. Do something on
impulse. Be spontaneous. If you suddenly feel inspired to do
something that's out of your usual routine and takes you out
of your comfort zone, just do it.

Heart-centred meditation

The word 'courage' comes from the French word *coeur*, which means 'heart'. Courage is a state of the heart. It is the ability to do what feels right, even if it scares you.

Breathe into your heart. Keep yourself calm and focused by taking heart-centred breaths. Place your hand on your heart and visualize breathing in and out of that heart space.

Always remember you are braver than you believe, stronger than you seem, and smarter than you think.

As Christopher Robin said to Winnie the Pooh.

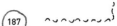

Lighten up

Instead or reading, watching or listening to the news or social media, start your days with a good sitcom episode or podcast.

Favourite sitcoms or podcasts

....

....

....

....

....

....

....

....

....

....

Remember

- What you think influences what you do and don't do. It's also true that what you do influences what you think.

- Energy spent on avoidance and escape could be better spent on thinking about what you can do – not what you think you can't do.

- Each time you take a small step outside your comfort zone, you widen your thoughts and beliefs about what you're capable of doing.

- What could feel impossible in one big leap, becomes a lot more doable as a series of smaller steps.

- CBT calls the step-by-step process 'graded exposure.' Exposure involves gradually doing the thing that you find stressful until you feel comfortable with each step. Think of it as carrying out an experiment: you're trying out new ways of behaving and seeing what happens.

- When the focus is on learning and improving, you're more likely to be calmer than if you think you have to get it right.

- Use your courage. This means accepting your fears and then working out a series of steps to work past them and achieve your goal.

- When you need courage and confidence, read one of your affirmations. It will give you reassurance that you can make it through a difficult situation.

- Focus on the benefits, not the difficulties. Instead of thinking about how hard something is, think about what you'll get out of it.

- Picture everything going well. Imagine that everything will work out. Visualize it.

- Minor setbacks and frustrating moments are habit killers; they give you an excuse to give up. For those 'what the hell moments', instead of giving up, think about and focus on what you have achieved in establishing your new good habit. Know that you can always take up where you left off, tomorrow.

Chapter 7
Emotions

Emotions and thoughts

Think of a time when you were pleased. What thoughts went through your mind?

Situation:

Thoughts:

Think of a time when you were angry. What thoughts went through your mind?

Situation:

Thoughts:

Think of a time when you felt guilty. What thoughts went through your mind?

Situation:

Thoughts:

Think of a time when you felt disappointed. What thoughts went through your mind?

Situation:

Thoughts:

Think of a time when you regretted something. What thoughts went through your mind?

Situation:

Thoughts:

Think of a time when you felt jealous. What thoughts went through your mind?

Situation:

Thoughts:

Let's not forget that the little emotions are the great captains of our lives and we obey them without realizing it.

Vincent Van Gogh

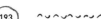

How it works

Thinking straight

I've just realized that the physical feelings for anger and excitement are the same. What's that about?

Yes, anger and excitement have the same physical feelings: rapid shallow breathing, increased heartbeat, stomach flipping over, tense ness, trembling.

What differentiates anger and excitement from each other are thoughts and behaviour.

Is it just me, or does everyone find it difficult to think in helpful, positive ways when they feel angry, guilty, disappointed, jealous etc.?

It's not just you! For all of us, the part of the brain (the amygdala) that's triggered when strong emotions arise (when we feel wronged, offended or threatened, ignored, embarrassed, humiliated etc.) is different from the part of the brain (the neo-cortex) that operates in rational and reasonable ways.

This means that when we feel strong emotions such as anger, jealousy humiliation etc, it's easy to be unreasonable and illogical because the anger has taken over our rational mind. Our ability to think in a clear, calm rational way has been switched off. It's as if a wall has come down and we're behind it.

Thoughts and emotions

Rumours have been going around the workplace that redundancies are soon going to be announced. Ali, Nik and Sara each have different thoughts about the possibility of losing their jobs.

Look at the three different interpretations below. Which emotions do you think are triggered by each of the different ways of thinking?

Nik: Oh dear, I'm sure they'll want to get rid of me. I'm not the best at this job - there're others they'll want to keep on.

Resignation, Bitterness, Hope, Anger, Anxiety, Optimism

Ali: I think I'll make a list of contacts, job agencies and similar companies and see what the job possibilities are right now.

Resignation, Bitterness, Hope, Anger, Anxiety, Optimism

Sara: It's not fair It's bound to be me. I'm going fight against this. I'll tell them they can't make me redundant.

Resignation, Bitterness, Hope, Anger, Anxiety, Optimism

The three parts of emotions

Emotions are communications from your brain, prompting you to do or not to do something.

Emotions are made up of three parts: thoughts, physical feelings and behaviour.

In any one situation, there's no one specific order in which the aspects of an emotion occur, but any one aspect can affect the others. What you think can affect how you physically feel. It can also alter how you behave. Equally, what you do – how you behave – can affect how you feel and what you think.

Although all emotions are made up of three aspects, cognitive therapy maintains that your emotions are strongly influenced by what you think.

Situation:

You come home to discover that the heating has broken down. Again.

Thoughts:

Oh my God! Not again. Why is this happening? It's not fair. I've had enough of this!

Physical reaction:

Tense muscles, heartrate increased and rapid breathing.

Behavioural reaction:

Throw your bag down, hard.

Emotion:

Anger.

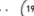

What might be the emotion, physical feelings, thoughts and behavioural responses for you in each of these situations?

Situation

A test, exam or interview.

Thoughts:

Physical reaction:

Behavioural reaction:

Emotion:

Situation:

You get the job, place on the course, the flat or the house.

Thoughts:

Physical reaction:

Behavioural reaction:

Emotion:

Situation:

The film/ meal/ party is cancelled.

Thoughts:

Physical reaction:

Behavioural reaction:

Emotion:

How it works

The positive intentions of 'negative' emotions

Why do we have emotions?

Emotions are your mind and body's way of communicating with you. They're prompting you to take positive, helpful action in response to something that has, is, or could happen. All emotions have a positive intent. 'Negative' emotions are only negative if you respond with negative thoughts and behaviour.

Imagine, for example, that you had to pull out of going to an important event with a friend. You feel guilty. You may think: 'I've let her down. I can tell she's upset and worried about going on her own. I feel bad.' Guilt, like *all* emotions, has a positive intent.

What can possibly be good or positive about feeling guilty?

The positive intent of guilt is to prompt you to recognize your wrongdoing and to think about what you could do to put right or make up for what you did wrong. And then do it.

If, though, when you feel guilty you simply wallow in your guilt, or try to suppress or deny how you feel, or even make up for your wrongdoing in inappropriate ways, then your thoughts and actions (or inaction) remain negative. Those thoughts and actions or inaction are not helpful.

OK. What about feeling anxious or frightened? How can those emotions be positive?

Fear is a clear example of an emotion that has a positive purpose: to protect you; to prompt you to fight or flight. Anxiety also has a positive purpose. Anxiety about an exam, for example, can motivate you to focus, to cut out all distractions and revise. Anxiety only becomes negative if it so overwhelms you that you're unable to think clearly enough to do the revision.

So, the problem is, when we experience a 'negative' emotion, we often reinforce it with unhelpful, negative thoughts and behaviour. Is that right?

Yes. Take, for example, regret. The positive intent of regret is to prompt you to learn from and avoid making a similar mistake in future. Regret is only negative if you become stuck in negative thoughts, self-blame and inaction. But that's not the emotion that is negative, it's your thinking and lack of positive action!

The positive intention of 'negative' emotions acts in the same way as the positive intention of physical pain. If you touch something really hot, the pain makes you pull away fast. It feels bad, but the positive intention of that pain is to protect you. It's the same with emotional pain; it can prompt you to take action – positive action.

Positive intentions

What do you think might be the positive purpose of:

1. **Anger: the strong feeling, the sense of injustice, in response to the notion that you or someone else has been wronged?**

    a) To motivate you to improve your situation.
    b) To put right a wrong.
    c) To steer clear of the person or thing.

2. **Envy: feeling resentful because someone else has something you don't?**

    a) To motivate you to improve your situation.
    b) To put right a wrong.
    c) To steer clear of the person or thing.

3. **Disgust: a strong aversion, a feeling of revulsion or loathing for something or someone?**

    a) To motivate you to improve your situation.
    b) To put right a wrong.
    c) To steer clear of the person or thing.

(Answers at the back of the book.)

How it works

Emotions and moods

What's the difference between an emotion and a mood?

Emotions are things that tend to come and go quite quickly. Emotions such as anger, surprise and joy are specific reactions to specific events: anger that your flight has been cancelled, surprise that you were given a discount on something you've bought, joy at the news of a new baby in the family.

Moods are longer lasting but less specific, less intense, and not so likely to be triggered by a particular event. A mood is a more general feeling such as apathy, sadness or contentment that lasts for a longer time: hours or days.

Emotions are more varied than moods; whilst we can have a wide range of different emotions, moods are more generalized: a good mood, a bad mood, a sad mood.

Emotions are sharper and more short-lived and they are directed at or are about something. You may feel irritated by something specific; having just missed the train for example. But a mood can make it more likely that you will feel an emotion and when this happens, the emotion may have the same character as the mood. For example you may be in an irritable mood, meaning you are easily irritated by missing the train.

So my emotions and thoughts can be influenced by my moods?

Yes, your emotions and the thoughts that go with them can be influenced by the mood you're in. If you're in a bad or sad mood, it's easy to interpret things in a way that reflects that mood.

Being in a bad mood makes you more prone to cognitive distortions such as jumping to conclusions, tunnel thinking, blaming etc.

Understanding the nature of moods and emotions can help you to see that the suspicion, frustration, disappointment, anxiety etc. you are feeling may well be influenced or heightened by a mood you were feeling before an event occurred.

What puts people in a bad or sad mood?

Being tired, hungry, having had too much to drink, stress etc. These are times and situations when negative unhelpful thoughts are easily triggered, as you won't have as much control over your thoughts and emotions.

When you're in a bad mood

Complete this sentence: If I'm in a bad or sad mood, to divert my thoughts and lift my mood it would help if I ...

☐ Eat: If I haven't eaten in a while my blood sugar may be low and I need to eat.

☐ Sleep: If I'm tired it's difficult to focus and stresses feel way worse.

☐ Change my surroundings: Go for a walk or a run. A cycle ride or swim.

☐ Listen to uplifting music: Sing and dance to music.

☐ Read a book, watch a film: A favourite book or film – something familiar that I know I'll enjoy.

Just be nice

Each week, do one of these things. Make a conscious effort to:

☐ Say 'Thank you'. Say it a lot!

☐ Stop moaning, complaining or criticizing for just three days.

☐ Don't be annoying. Avoid doing the things you know annoy the person or people you live with or work with.

☐ Hold your tongue. Wait before speaking or writing when you are irritated, annoyed or angry.

☐ Look for the good in someone you don't like.

☐ Share, even if you don't really want to.

☐ Do the task no one else wants to do.

☐ Don't leave others waiting for you. Be on time.

☐ Let someone else have their way.

☐ Respond to emails and texts. Don't leave others waiting even if you have to say, 'I'll get right back to you ASAP'. People like to know they're not being ignored.

☐ Smile more often.

Cloud-spotting meditation

Try a spot of cloud spotting. From the fluffy cumulus that form on a sunny day, to the higher level cirrocumulus clouds there's an endless variety of clouds that appear in the sky and their fleeting beauty remind you that all things – emotions and moods – will pass.

I believe your atmosphere and your surroundings create a mind state for you.

Theophilus London

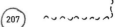

Emotions

Below is a list of emotions. Put a tick next to the words that you usually use to describe feelings.

☐ Adore	☐ Eager	☐ Loathe
☐ Afraid	☐ Elated	☐ Love
☐ Alarmed	☐ Embarrassed	☐ Miserable
☐ Amused	☐ Enraged	☐ Outraged
☐ Angry	☐ Envious	☐ Panic
☐ Anticipating	☐ Exasperated	☐ Passionate
☐ Anxious	☐ Excited	☐ Peturbed
☐ Ashamed	☐ Exhilarated	☐ Pity
☐ Awesome	☐ Fear	☐ Proud
☐ Bewildered	☐ Fond	☐ Regret
☐ Bored	☐ Frustrated	☐ Resent
☐ Compassionate	☐ Grateful	☐ Sad
☐ Contemptuous	☐ Guilty	☐ Scared
☐ Confused	☐ Happy	☐ Seething
☐ Curious	☐ Hate	☐ Shocked
☐ Delighted	☐ Hopeful	☐ Shy
☐ Despairing	☐ Horrified	☐ Spiteful
☐ Disappointed	☐ Hostile	☐ Surprised
☐ Dismayed	☐ Humiliated	☐ Suspicious
☐ Disgusted	☐ Irritated	☐ Troubled
☐ Distraught	☐ Joyful	☐ Terrified
☐ Distressed	☐ Jubilant	☐ Worried
☐ Dread	☐ Like	

Definitions

Look up some of the words you've ticked in a dictionary or on
a dictionary website. Do you agree with the definitions? Does
the dictionary's definition of the word 'frustrated' for example,
reflect how you feel when *you* use that word?

Word:

Definition:

Word:

Definition:

Word:

Definition:

Sizes of emotions

What words for feelings do you usually use? If you use the word 'angry' you will find that 'frustrated' and 'enraged' are similar. The obvious difference between these words is that they describe different levels of intensity of anger.

What about the word 'embarrassed'? Are there situations where the word 'humiliated' might be more appropriate? Could there be words that are closer to what you are actually feeling in some situations?

Put the following words in order according to their intensity:

like, adore, love, fond, devoted, cherish, affection, desire, care for

sad, disappointed, let down, unhappy, hurt, distressed, dissatisfied

irritated, enraged, angry, furious, annoyed, seething, aggravated, put out, perturbed

jubilant, thrilled, exhilarated, amused, cheerful, delighted, glad, contented, pleased, happy, satisfied, euphoric, ecstatic, elated

anxious, uneasy, worried, bewildered, confused, lost, unsure, vague, mixed up

Alternative words

If you're like most people, you probably don't stop to think and choose the words to describe your emotions. Most of us are in the habit of using the same dozen or so words to describe feeling mad, sad, glad or scared.

The words you use to describe your experience *become* your experience. If you think or say 'I'm devastated' you're going to produce a different effect than if you say, 'I'm very disappointed'.

The words you use can magnify an emotion or soften it.

Of course, there are times when you do feel furious or devastated. But it's easy to habitually use the same strong words for different situations. Just changing the habitual words you use to describe what you're feeling, can help shift your thoughts and feelings.

Identify the words you use most often to describe emotions and find a new word for each one.

Often-used emotion words:

Alternative words:

New words for emotions

Have you ever felt something but not got a word to describe it? Often, words do exist to describe those feelings, they're just not English words! Tick any of the emotions you've felt.

- ☐ *Schadenfreude* (German) The pleasure derived from someone else's pain.
- ☐ *Firgun* (Hebrew) Saying nice things to someone simply to make them feel good.
- ☐ *Gigil* (Filipino) The urge to pinch or squeeze something that is unbearably cute.
- ☐ *Litost* (Czech) A state of torment created by the sudden sight of one's own misery.
- ☐ *Pena ajena* (Mexican Spanish) The embarrassment you feel watching someone else's humiliation.
- ☐ *Iktsuarpok* (Inuit) The feeling of anticipation when you're waiting for someone to show up.
- ☐ *Fremdschämen* (German) Being embarrassed for someone who should be but isn't.
- ☐ *Tartle* (Scots) The panicky hesitation just before you have to introduce someone whose name you can't quite remember.
- ☐ *Gezelligheid* (Dutch) The comfort and coziness of being at home, with friends, with loved ones or general togetherness.
- ☐ *Mudita* (Sanskrit) Revelling in someone else's joy.
- ☐ *Sitzfleisch* (German) The ability to persevere through hard or boring tasks (literally 'sit meat').

Invent your own emotions

What words would you invent for the feelings that come with these situations?

1. The realization you've forgotten a friend's birthday.

2. Waking up knowing you have something really good happening that day.

3. Listening to someone who can only talk about themselves.

4. The feeling you have just as the plane takes off.

5. The feeling you have when someone else has put crockery or saucepans back in the wrong cupboard.

Write down your own situations and invented words for the feelings that go with them

Situations:

Invented emotion words:

Identifying your strongest thoughts and feelings

Rating thoughts and emotions can help you identify what's really bothering you in a situation.

Situation:

A friend lets you know that he's cancelling your evening together; he's just been offered a ticket to see his favourite band.

Thoughts:

Oh great. Now I'm not going out tonight. 7

This isn't the first time he's done this. 4

I'd have liked to have seen that band, too. 6

No one ever offers me any nice last-minute surprises. 8

Emotions:

Disappointed 7

Annoyed 5

Jealous 9

Lonely 9

Write down some situations that you have experienced.
Include the thoughts and emotions that you experienced. If
you write down more than one thought or emotion, identify the
'strongest' thought by rating the strength of your thoughts and
emotions on a scale of 1–10.

Situation:

Thoughts:

Emotions:

Draw a circle round the strongest one. This will ensure that you
focus on the thoughts and feelings that affect you the most.

Feed the other tiger

Once there lived an old man who kept many different kinds of animals. Two tigers that lived together in one cage particularly intrigued his grandson. The tigers had different temperaments; one was calm and self-controlled whilst the other was unpredictable, aggressive, violent, and vicious.

'Do they ever fight, Grandfather?' asked the boy.

'Occasionally, yes they do,' admitted the old man.

'And which one wins?'

'Well, that depends on which one I feed the most.'

Being able to manage your emotions depends in part on how much you 'feed' a particular emotion. No matter what the emotion, there's always more than one way to think and respond.

Responsible thoughts

Think of the occasions when you have felt guilty, angry, upset, jealous or disappointed. Did you blame someone else for feeling the way you did? At any point did you think 'You/he/she/they made me feel...?'

Rephrase this. Saying, 'He made me angry' blames the other person for how you feel. On the other hand, saying, 'I am feeling angry' is taking responsibility for feeling that way.

When you take responsibility for how you feel then, like anything else that belongs to you, you get to choose what to do about how you feel.

Complete the sentences below.

1. They've embarrassed me. I'm:

2. You've deceived me. I feel:

3. She made me feel that I've done something wrong. I feel:

4. He's disappointed me. I am:

5. They made me feel really small. I feel:

6. He made me feel bad about what I said. I feel:

7. She's upset me. I feel:

Letting go meditation

Remember a time when you experienced a difficult situation. Maybe a friend let you down, someone humiliated you, you made a mistake or you embarrassed yourself. You may still be feeling hurt, disappointed, jealous or angry. Whatever the feeling, breathe it in as hot, heavy, polluted smoke. Breathe in for a count of five.

Breathe out to the count of five. Breathe out the hot, heavy smoke of hurt, guilt, regret or anger. Feel the sense of release and surrender that arises. Don't analyse what you're doing. Don't try to figure it out. Don't justify it.

Simply breathe in this way for between five and ten breaths. Breathe in the heavy, hot smoke of your suffering and breathe out to let it go.

Emotional triggers

We all have emotional triggers – specific events that provoke an automatic emotional reaction. In fact, emotional triggers usually cause us to overreact – to respond more strongly than is necessary or appropriate.

Learning to recognize your own personal triggering situations can be a helpful step towards changing your automatic reactions.

You can't predict every situation but there are some that you know will set you off. What can suddenly make you scared and frightened? What immediately frustrates you? What sort of situations always leave you feeling disappointed and resentful? What do you know for certain will leave you feeling guilty or humiliated?

☐ Computer not doing what you want it to do

☐ Forgetting to phone your parents

☐ Someone else's dangerous driving

☐ Being ignored

☐ Not understanding

☐ Being left out

☐ Having to wait for someone

☐ Traffic hold ups

☐ Too much to do in too little time

☐ Being lied to

☐ Being told what to do and how to do it

☐ Uncooperative children

☐ When you're blamed, judged or criticized

☐ Feeling unwelcome

☐ Experiencing unfairness

☐ Feeling uncertain

Other situations:

☐

☐

☐

☐

Identify emotional triggers

Often, you won't identify an emotional trigger until after it's pulled. Next time you have a strong emotional reaction to something, write it down. Note the emotion and what happened to trigger the emotion.

Notice your thoughts: 'How dare he!' or 'Oh no! I feel awful' for example. Notice your physical feelings: maybe you feel tense, are breathing quickly, or can feel your heart thumping.

Notice your behaviour: perhaps you are becoming tearful or raising your voice and snapping.

Triggering event:

Emotions:

Thoughts:

Physical feelings:

Behaviour:

Label the emotion

Labelling your emotion means simply saying to yourself, 'This feels like (for example) disappointment'.

Just notice the feeling without reacting. Say something accepting to yourself, like, 'Ok, I'm feeling resentful right now', 'Yes, this is sadness', or 'I'm angry and that's ok'. Just acknowledging and accepting your feelings will increase your ability not to be overwhelmed or overreact.

Before you attempt to change anything, just be aware of the emotion, and the thoughts and physical feelings that accompany it.

Remember

- The part of the brain (the amygdala) that's triggered when strong emotions arise is different from the part of the brain (the neo-cortex) that operates in rational and reasonable ways.

- This means that when strong emotions are triggered, it's easy to be unreasonable and illogical because the anger has taken over your rational mind. Your ability to think in a clear, calm rational way has been switched off.

Engage your brain

As soon as you notice that you're reacting emotionally – thinking unhelpful thoughts and feeling tense, breathing quickly, raising your voice – you need to access the rational thinking part of your brain so that you can respond in a conscious, helpful way; a way that doesn't make things worse.

☐ Breathe: breathe out for longer than you breathe in.

☐ Stop breathing for five seconds (to 'reset' your breath).

☐ Next, breathe in slowly for three seconds and then breathe out more slowly – for five seconds.

☐ Continue focusing on breathing in to a slow count of three and out to a slow count of five for a minute. Be aware that it's the out breath that will slow everything down.

Imagine yourself as a pot of water about to boil over. Nothing will instantly cool you off completely, but taking a minute to breathe and separate yourself from the heat source will keep things from getting beyond your control.

Just having to think about and count those three seconds then five seconds can help engage your rational, reasoning brain. It won't completely dispel the emotion – disappointment, anxiety or frustration – but it can bring you to a calmer place so that you can think straight.

You can also engage the rational, reasoning part of your brain in other ways:

☐ Recite the alphabet

☐ Count to 50

☐ Recite the alphabet backwards

☐ Count backwards from 50

Emotions say hurry. Wisdom says wait.

Anon

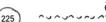

Remember

- All emotions have a positive intent. 'Negative' emotions are only negative if you respond with negative thoughts and behaviour.

- Emotions and the thoughts that go with them can be influenced by the mood you're in. If you're in a bad or sad mood, it's easy to interpret things in a way that reflects that mood.

- The words you use to describe your experience *become* your experience. If you think or say 'I'm devastated' you're going to produce a different effect than if you say 'I'm very disappointed'.

- Just changing the habitual words you use to describe what you're feeling can help shift your thoughts and feelings.

- When you take responsibility for how you feel then, like anything else that belongs to you, you get to choose what to do about how you feel.

- Learning to recognize your own personal triggering situations can be a helpful step towards changing your automatic reactions.

- As soon as you notice that you're reacting emotionally, try to access the rational thinking part of your brain so that you can respond in a conscious, helpful way, a way that doesn't make things worse.

Chapter 8

Conceptualizing

How it works

Conceptualizing

Conceptualizing involves looking at each aspect of a situation (the event, your thoughts, physical feelings and behaviour) and instead of them being jumbled up in your mind, organizing them in a way that can help you to see any connections between those thoughts, feelings and behaviour.

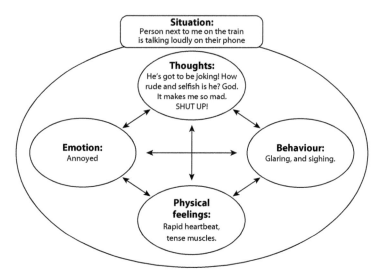

Notice how the arrows in the conceptualization go both ways: thoughts, feelings and behaviours feed into and strengthen each other.

In the next example, one aspect of the situation (the thoughts) has changed. Notice how this has now changed the rest of the dynamic.

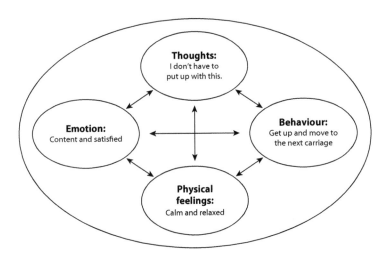

Thoughts:
I don't have to put up with this.

Emotion:
Content and satisfied

Behaviour:
Get up and move to the next carriage

Physical feelings:
Calm and relaxed

Change one thing

For each of the two situations, write in the emotion, physical feelings and behaviour that would be likely to follow the new thoughts.

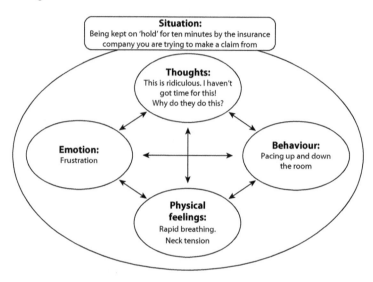

Situation:
Being kept on 'hold' for ten minutes by the insurance company you are trying to make a claim from

Thoughts:
This is ridiculous. I haven't got time for this!
Why do they do this?

Emotion:
Frustration

Behaviour:
Pacing up and down the room

Physical feelings:
Rapid breathing.
Neck tension

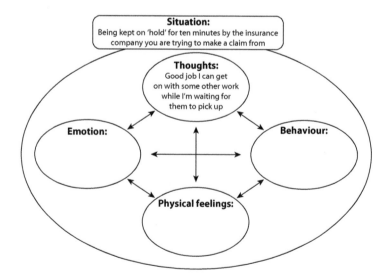

Situation:
Being kept on 'hold' for ten minutes by the insurance company you are trying to make a claim from

Thoughts:
Good job I can get on with some other work while I'm waiting for them to pick up

Emotion:

Behaviour:

Physical feelings:

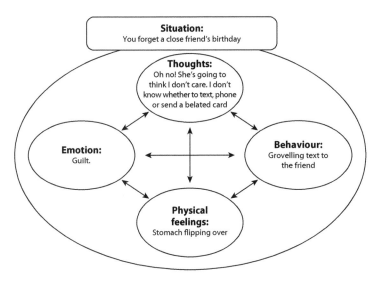

Situation:
You forget a close friend's birthday

Thoughts:
Oh no! She's going to think I don't care. I don't know whether to text, phone or send a belated card

Emotion:
Guilt.

Behaviour:
Grovelling text to the friend

Physical feelings:
Stomach flipping over

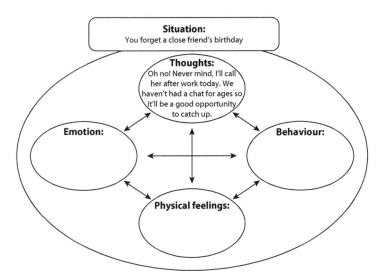

Situation:
You forget a close friend's birthday

Thoughts:
Oh no! Never mind, I'll call her after work today. We haven't had a chat for ages so it'll be a good opportunity to catch up.

Emotion:

Behaviour:

Physical feelings:

Conceptualization map

Create your own conceptualization map for a recent difficult event.

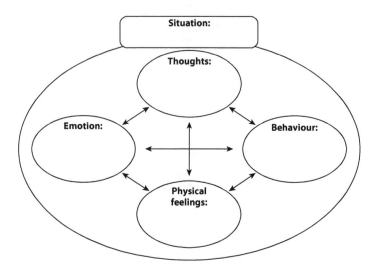

Now keep the same situation but write an alternative for the 'Thoughts' circle. Then complete the map.

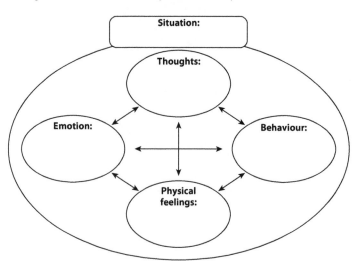

Next time you've experienced a strong emotion (for example anger, joy, guilt, embarrassment), try to identify each aspect – the physical feelings, the thoughts and behaviour. There are blank conceptualization maps at the back of the book for you to use.

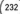

Reasons to use conceptualization maps

Conceptualization maps provide and show a structure to difficulties and problems in any one situation. They can:

o Help you to see the whole picture: make the connection between your thoughts about something and the way you're feeling and behaving.

o Show you how situations, thoughts, physical feelings and emotions affect each other and can lead to difficulties being maintained or even increased.

o Help identify the key 'problem maintaining' thoughts and behaviours of a situation.

o Help you to see, in any one situation, which aspect is most easily altered to positively change the other aspects.

o Allow you to try out different possibilities; try changing different aspects.

Good habit

Go with the flow

Think of the times you've been so absorbed in what you were doing that time passed without you realizing. It could've been a good book or a film, doing a puzzle, a meal out with friends or playing a sport. Whatever it was, as you did it, no other thoughts entered your mind because you were completely caught up in what you were doing; you didn't even notice the time that was passing.

This state of mind is known as 'flow'. When your mind is in a state of flow it's so engaged that it's difficult for your mind to wander off and there's no room for difficult, worrying thoughts to find their way into your head.

What do you like doing? What activities can you dip into for ten minutes or immerse yourself in for an hour?

☐ Listening to music or playing an instrument

☐ Reading a novel

☐ Watching a film

☐ Doing a puzzle – a crossword or sudoku

☐ Playing a computer game

☐ Yoga, Tai Chi, Pilates

☐ A game of tennis, badminton or football

☐ Housework

☐ Drawing, painting

☐ Gardening, cooking and baking

☐

☐

☐

The times I feel most alive are when I'm caught up in something that makes me forget myself. Art. Work. People. Nature.

Donald Miller

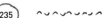

Good news

At the end of each day, identify three small positive things that happened. You'll soon find yourself actively looking for things to appreciate and, after a while, it will become a habit. A positive habit.

For positive, inspiring news, ideas and stories, go to these websites.

http://www.dailygood.org/

http://www.huffingtonpost.com/good-news/

http://www.goodnewsnetwork.org/

https://www.positive.news/

http://www.sunnyskyz.com/

Favourite headlines:

☐

☐

☐

☐

☐

Give yourself a medal

> This is to certify that
>
> ....
>
> has completed the
>
> ## CBT Good Habit Journal

Congratulations! You've come to the end of the journal. Use this page to record what you have learned and achieved from this book.

Success comes in cans not in can'ts.

Anon

How to eat an elephant

Think you can't eat an elephant?

That it's too big a task?

You don't know until you have tried

You have to prepare and plan for it

You have to be hungry for it

You need to be committed and really put your mind to it

You need to get the measure of what you are dealing with

It's an unpredictable animal that requires careful handling

Clear your head

Focus

Concentrate on the task in hand

Sit with it for a while

Contemplate

Do you have the right tools and equipment?

Do you need instruction?

Do you need more learning?

Do you need more experience?

Do you need a mentor?

Do you need an expert with the right skills and experience

Do you need someone by your side along the way?

Don't be discouraged by people telling you it can't be done.
It can

It's not going to be easy. No one said it would be

If you want easy this is not for you

It's going to challenge you but you will grow from the
experience

Think outside the box when you need to

Be creative. There is more than one way to do this

The simplest way may not be the right one

Don't exhaust yourself trying

Accept setbacks along the way. They happen

Break it down into smaller pieces

Don't give up

Stop and regroup when you need to

Find a new or different way

Be patient and stay connected

It will require sacrifice

It's going to be worth it

Be brave

Be courageous

Take the risk

You won't regret it

It may protest

It may roar

It may try to run away from you

Wait and take stock

Be patient

Let negative thoughts come and go. They will pass

Try again

Each step will take you closer

You *can* do it

Use your imagination and creativity

You can overcome any obstacles it puts in your way

Determination will see you though

Failure is not an option

Face it head on

Look it in the eye

Don't waver

It may take several attempts

You may have to leave it a while and return later

You will come across parts that are tough

Chew them up and spit them out

You are going to reach the sweeter meat

It will be exquisite

Enjoy the journey and achievements along the way

You have travelled far to get there.

Once it is in your grasp

Feel the exhilaration

Don't overfill your plate

Share your bounty with others

Savour each bite

It is the taste of your success

Remember...

If you can do this you can do anything

After all, elephants can't fly but you can.

Julie Finch 2017

Answers

Chapter 2
Spot the cognitive distortions

1 b, c, d, e and f; 2 b and e; 3 a; 4 b, c and d; 5 c and d; 6 f

Chapter 3
Lateral thinking: the cake

Solution 1: Use two cuts to divide the cake into four equal pieces (quarters). For the third cut, cut the cake in half, horizontally. Some pieces may not have any icing, but their size will be equal.

Solution 2: As in the first solution, use two cuts to divide the cake into four equal pieces (quarters). Then, stack the four pieces on top of each other and use a third cut to cut all four pieces in two.

Lateral thinking: the bus stop

The old lady of course! After helping the old lady into the car, you can give your keys to your friend, and wait with your perfect partner for the bus.

Chapter 5
True or false?

1. No. it isn't; 2. They can see almost as well as humans. However, at night, their ears are more important than their eyes – they use a special sonar system called 'echolocation,' meaning they find things using echoes; 3. Goldfish have a memory of up to five months; 4. Some all-white cats suffer from congenital deafness caused by a degeneration of the inner ear; 5. Nowhere in the New Testament does it say there were three – this was the number of gifts that were given to Jesus (gold, frankincense and myrrh). In the book of Matthew

(Chapter 2, Verse 1) it says: 'Now when Jesus was born in Bethlehem of Judaea in the days of Herod the king, behold, there came wise men from the east to Jerusalem; 6. The diuretic effect is mild and offset by the liquid in the caffeinated drink; 7. While you might not be using every bit of your brain at all times, you do use your entire brain over the course of the day. Feeling like someone isn't living up to his or her full potential is a different matter, but that still doesn't mean they aren't using their entire brain each day; 8. It is not that the hair and fingernails are growing, but that the surrounding skin retracts as it becomes dehydrated, and pulls away from the hair shafts and nail beds. The hair and fingernails are not affected by the lack of moisture and do not shrink, which can make it seem as if they had grown; 9. Alcohol dilates the blood vessels near the skin giving the impression of warmth but actually, drinking alcohol lowers the core temperature of your body; 10. How long it takes to form a habit depends on several things – mainly, the habit being formed, the individual and their motivation and reasons for changing.

Chapter 6
Graded exposure

1.1. Choose one drawer or cupboard to sort out.

1.2. Take out everything from chosen drawer or cupboard and put onto the table

1.3. Take out broken, chipped or cracked things and put in a box.

1.4. Put back in the cupboard/drawer those items – crockery, pans, cutlery etc. – that I use often.

1.5. Put what's left – unwanted items – into a box.

1.6. Take unwanted items to charity shop.

1.7. Repeat the process with another drawer or cupboard on another day.

2.1 Go to the open day and meet the tutor in the room where the class will take place.

2.2 Before the course begins, go to the college with a friend and have a coffee in the café.

2.3 Before the course begins, go to the college on a busy day on my own and have a coffee in the café.

2.4 Phone a friend for encouragement on my way to the first class.

2.5 Go to the first class – be the first to arrive.

Chapter 7
Positive intentions

1. B; 2. A; 3. C

Negative/Alternative thought record

Situation:

Negative thought:

How much do you believe this thought on a scale of 1-10?

What evidence do you have to support this thought?

Alternative thought:

What evidence do you have to support this alternative view?

How much do you believe the alternative thought on a scale of 1-10)?

Negative/Alternative thought record

Situation:

Negative thought:

How much do you believe this thought on a scale of 1-10?

What evidence do you have to support this thought?

Alternative thought:

What evidence do you have to support this alternative view?

How much do you believe the alternative thought on a scale of 1-10)?

Conceptualization maps

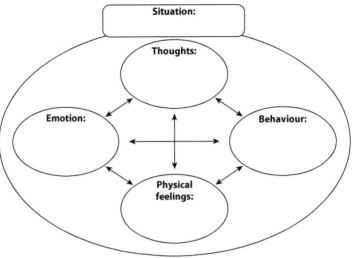

Situation:

Thoughts:

Emotion:

Behaviour:

Physical feelings:

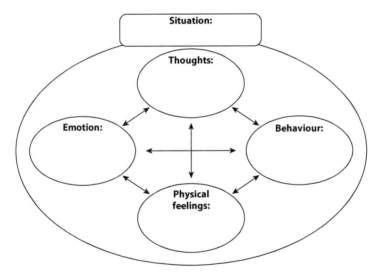

Situation:

Thoughts:

Emotion:

Behaviour:

Physical feelings:

Conceptualization maps

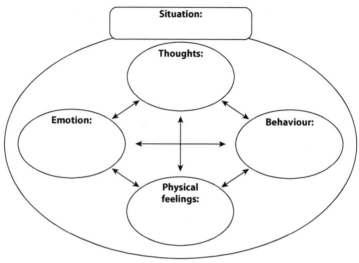

Situation:

Thoughts:

Emotion:

Behaviour:

Physical feelings:

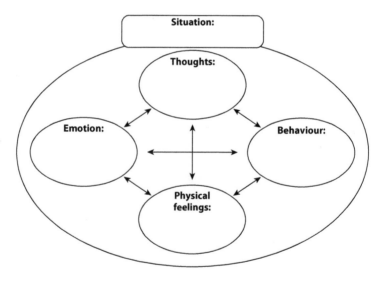

Situation:

Thoughts:

Emotion:

Behaviour:

Physical feelings: